TRANSFORM
YOUR BODY
TRANSFORM
YOUR LIFE

MASTER YOUR MIND & BODY
TO BE IN THE SHAPE OF
YOUR LIFE, FOR LIFE

AKASH VAGHELA

R3THINK PRESS

Illustrations by Suraj Sodha.

Photography credits:
p x by Simon Howard
pp x, xi, 27, 196, 200, 210, 223 by Ben Mark
pp x, xi, 106, 196, 200, 207, 221, 224 by Shyam Kotecha
p 223 by Jayesh Pankhania
p 223 by Noel Daganta
p 224 by Samuel Githegi

PRAISE

'If you want a quick-fix 12-week plan, don't read this book. This is for those of you who want a real lifelong transformation – inside and out. A refreshingly honest book for the fitness industry.'

— **Jason Ferruggia**, transformation coach and host of the Renegade Radio podcast

'Staying in great shape in the long run takes more than simply eating less and moving more. It requires a fundamental rewiring of how you think and act on a daily basis. If you would love to be a brand-new fit and vital individual then this book will be your roadmap for how to achieve it.'

— **Dr John Demartini**, international bestselling author, educator and consultant

'Akash has delivered a superb book dedicated to the greater good of your life. It's as much a manual for the spirit as it is for the physical, and it is packed with superb ideas and life observations that reject the quick fix and reveal the secrets of a life journey. Its author has leant on his own life experiences, and in so doing, has produced an inspiring read, with fresh insights and accessible lessons to achieve the shape of your life, for life.'

— **Michael Hayman**, MBE, co-author of *Mission: How the best in business break through*

'If you're ready to break the dieting cycle and transform for life, this book is what you need. Read it!'

— **Shona Vertue**, author and creator of the Vertue Method

'The way fitness is marketed, you'd never know there's a difference between short-term results and long-term transformations. Akash used to think that way, too – until he tried it, and it nearly broke him. That's when he realised that the biggest transformation is the one that takes place between your ears. *Transform Your Body, Transform Your Life* is an expert guide to making those big changes, from someone who's learned these lessons the hard way.'

— **Lou Schuler**, editorial director at the Personal Trainer Development Center

'This book transcends the fitness industry. The principles, methods and insights it contains can be applied in your business, your career and your relationships. It's a must-have for anyone in any industry.'

— **Phil Graham**, leading fitness educator and author of *Diabetic Muscle and Fitness Guide*

CONTENTS

INTRODUCTION 1

1 NEW BEGINNINGS 7

Four reasons for failure 7
Discovering your trigger 13
Overriding the chaos 17
The five-step process to real goals 20
Creating realistic expectations 24
The power of accountability 32
The five phases of your transformation journey 35
Your journey is your own 40
It's never just about the physical 40

2 PHASE ONE: CLEANING THE PALATE 43

Mastering the 3Ss 45
CTP accelerators 58
Managing decision fatigue 58
Installing non-negotiables 63
Mastering precursors 64
Does CTP ever end? 70
Summary 72

3 PHASE TWO: PROCESS 75

Ticking the boxes in five stages 75
The honeymoon period 77
The motivation dip 77
Gathered momentum 79

The precision dip 79
The grind 84
Process accelerators 89
The art of the buffer 90
Social stigma armoury 94
Hunger suppressors 97
Be a leader 98
Be an essentialist 100
Transformation checkpoint 110
Summary 111

4   PHASE THREE: CONSOLIDATION   113

Avoiding the rebound 116
Consolidation accelerators 121
Developing meal hygiene 122
Shifting from an aesthetic to performance mindset 128
Maintaining your accountability systems 129
Don't punish yourself 130
It gets easier every time 131
Mastering the tip of the mountain 136
Conquering consolidation 142
Summary 143

5   PHASE FOUR: INVESTMENT   145

A lesson in an auto rickshaw 145
What do you want? 147
Investment accelerators 152
Lifestyle management 152
Performance indicators 160
Health optimisation 162
Autoregulation 166
Minimum investment periods 174
Summary 183

6   PHASE FIVE: REWARD   185

What exactly is the reward phase?   186
Your unique lifestyle solution   187
Walking into the dream house   192
The evolving big why   197
Reward accelerators   201
Rebalancing priorities   201
Embracing new challenges   202
Recycling the journey   204
Pay your dues   211
Summary   212

7   BRINGING IT ALL TOGETHER   213

The three transformation keys   213
It's more than just the physical   215
Do it for yourself, but don't do it alone   216
Read in between the lines   217
You owe it to yourself   218

Afterword   225
RNT resources   229
References   231
RNT Glossary   233
Acknowledgements   237
The Author   241

I dedicate this book to those of you using the physical as the vehicle for the greater good in your life. I hope the benefits you experience allow you to do things you never dreamed of.

ARWINDER

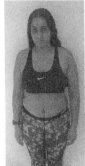 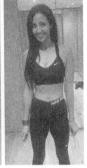

ADAM

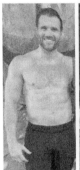 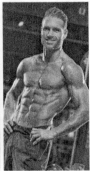

SUMETHA

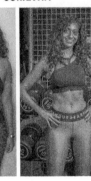

SHYAM

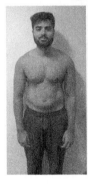 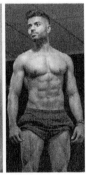

PUJA

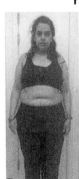 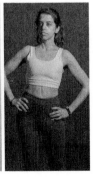

KEVIN

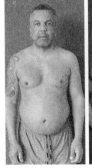 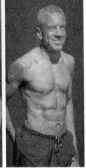

X

SHIV

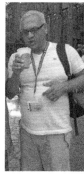

NINA

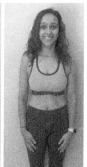

DIKSESH

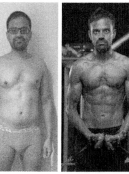

RANJANA

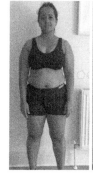

AKASH

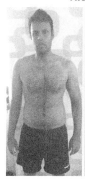

SANJEETA

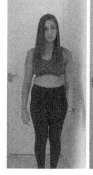

INTRODUCTION

Getting into shape is easy. You eat less and move more over a consistent period of time. Millions of people around the world are doing this every day. But staying in shape is a different ball game. That's the hard bit.

Why are so many people stuck in a dieting cycle for the rest of their lives? Why can't people maintain their weight after they lose it? Why is yo-yo dieting and rebounding so common? Why is the health and fitness industry worth billions of pounds[1] if no one is happy? Why are people not experiencing the results they desire?

This book explains why.

If you've fallen into the trap of dieting and gaining all the weight back, I don't blame you. It's not your fault. The bigger problem in the health and fitness industry is the quick-fix short-term mindset geared towards *only* being in the shape of your life. Magazines and social media are fuelling this with new four-week blitzes, eight-week shape-ups and twelve-week plans coming out every single day. While these plans can produce great results in the short term, what about the long term? What are you supposed to do once you get into shape? How can you translate a short-term change into a long-term transformation?

It's time for a paradigm shift, and it starts here. This book is designed to give you the blueprint for getting into the shape of your life *for* life.

---

1 IMARC Group (2019) 'Weight Management Market: Global industry trends, share, size, growth, opportunity and forecast 2019–2024'. www.imarcgroup.com

Before we dive into the concepts I'm going to share, it would be a good idea for me to give you some background. After all, why should you listen to me if you don't know where I'm coming from?

My career so far has been one of two halves. I started out as a personal trainer in 2010, where my sole focus was on helping busy people get into the best shape possible. This was my life for five years, and I was getting great results.

But then it all changed. In 2014, I decided to test myself and try my luck with competitive bodybuilding. After four months of hard dieting, I got into the shape of my life and won my first show. I felt more confident than ever, on top of the world, but that lasted only a few days. And I wasn't prepared for what came next.

Fast forward a couple of months, and I experienced the dreaded rebound. I was in worse shape than when I'd started. All the short-term benefits I'd experienced had quickly dissipated. I had no idea what to do, how to cope or how to react. I was lost.

In the aftermath of the rebound, I started to reflect on why this had happened. I realised that until 2014, I'd only ever cared about the process of getting *into* shape, both for myself and my clients. *I* was the person pushing quick-fix solutions. Once the classic 'after' picture was taken, in my mind the job was done. It's true. I wish I was lying.

In the two years that followed, I slowly got myself back on track. At the same time, I was beginning to understand the difference between those who get into shape and those who stay in shape. It had never been about the diet plan, training programme or supplement protocol. In the first five years of my career, that's all I cared about. It worked for a short-term change, but I learnt that for long-term transformation, I needed to go deeper.

Being lean and healthy for life means a fundamental internal rewiring. You can't only change what you put in your mouth, or how you train; you need to shift your entire identity, behaviour and mindset. You need to live by rules. It becomes more than just the physical; you need to think and act differently.

When starting RNT Fitness in 2017, I formalised my learnings into the five phases of the RNT Transformation Journey,[2] which is a step-by-step approach to enable you to get into the shape of your life, for life. Since this new beginning, my team and I have refined our methods to help transform thousands of busy people across more than twenty countries around the world. Before starting their journeys, they were in a similar position to the one I was in. They were fed up with quick fixes, yo-yoing and rebounds. They were tired of spinning their wheels with no long-term results to show for their hard work. They were frustrated with being unable to bridge the gap between a short-term change and a long-term transformation. You may be in that position too right now.

Life is different for my clients now. They've changed their paradigm. This book is going to teach you how to do the same. My aim is to take an initial change and use it as a stepping-stone to

---

2 One of the many things I love about RNT is 'RNT speak'. I define each RNT word and phrase throughout the book, but for ease of reference, I've also included a glossary at the end.

build a long-term lifestyle solution. This is my why. I've written this book to stop you making the same mistakes I made for years, with both myself and my clients.

My mission in the world is to help busy people use the physical as the vehicle to transform their lives. This book is part of that mission. As you go through the five phases of the transformation journey, the benefits you'll experience will transcend the physical. By mastering your body and rewiring your behaviour, identity and mindset, you will transform your life. You'll be more confident, focused and in control. You'll feel, look and perform at your best. You'll no longer have to worry about endless dieting, rebounding or yo-yoing. You'll push yourself to do more in all areas of life: relationships, career and health.

Be prepared, though – this book will ask a lot of you. It'll force you to question your actions and thought processes, and unlock a whole new level of self-awareness. It will take you a step closer to self-mastery as you continuously strive for improvement. Of course, it will be up to you to take action and apply the methodology, and it'll take trial and error before you get it right. Stick with it, though, because the payoff is extraordinary.

I will begin by addressing the core reasons why most people are failing to transform. I'll also discuss the underpinnings of a successful long-term transformation, and the hard questions you need to ask yourself before starting this journey. At some point, you're almost certain to have an aha moment. A light-bulb in your head will shine so brightly, you're likely to stop reading and take stock. I can't tell you when it'll happen or what it'll be, as each of you will have a different background and struggle. But you'll know it when it hits you.

At the beginning of this book, you will have seen a small selection of the clients we've worked with who've used their aha moments to achieve something great. Throughout the book, I'll tell some of their stories to inspire yours. If there's a story you'd like to hear more of, simply head to www.rntfit-ness.com/book-bonuses. You'll be able to read case studies, watch videos and listen to podcasts featuring these incredible people, and many more.

These clients have let go of their past, and are now shaping their future. I hope this book brings you the same, and I'm excited to begin the transformation journey together with you.

Are you ready?

1
NEW BEGINNINGS

FOUR REASONS FOR FAILURE

It's time for a new way of thinking. We need to question every belief we have been holding on to about body transformation. The multibillion-pound industry is brainwashing us, and it's doing an incredible job of it. Let's start by changing this, exploring the four reasons so many have failed in their pursuit of being in the shape of their life, for life.

I've been in the fortunate position to have read thousands of enquiries from prospective clients who are nearly at breaking point but are ready to try one more time to find something that works for them. In almost all cases, their failure to master their body has come as a result of:

1. A lack of perspective regarding the different milestones (death of the twelve-week plan)

2. A lack of knowledge of the long-term process (what do I do next?)

3. A lack of belief in what they can achieve and how (what and how?)

4. A lack of clear underpinnings to their journey (the why)

All four relate to the long-term journey they're on. To fix their mistakes, they require a change in thinking and approach. It's critical before we go through the five phases that you understand each problem and ask yourself if you've fallen victim to one (or all) of them.

DEATH OF THE TWELVE-WEEK PLAN

I'll admit it: I was guilty of being on the twelve-week transformation bandwagon for many of the early years of my career. It's sexy, it sells and it's an achievable timeframe for anyone wanting to see a change in their body. The problem is, that's all it does. It changes, it does not transform. It throws all your eggs into one basket and applies a singular focus to one goal, one date and one timeframe. That's why it works. It's also why it fails.

I'm all for creating deadlines, and twelve weeks is a great milestone for you to work towards. My problem is how you may perceive the twelve weeks. In the past, you may have said things such as:

- It's only twelve weeks

- Two weeks down, ten to go

- I'm at the halfway mark – six weeks to blast it

- Final week then I'm done

- I can't wait for the twelve weeks to be over

The issue is all in the language – the subconscious self-talk that after twelve weeks, it's all over. You're giving yourself permission to go back to your old habits, behaviours and practices after twelve weeks. That's why you often hear people say, 'Credit for losing the weight, but the hard bit is keeping it off.' It's why in my experience, over 90% of those who embark on twelve-week plans end up back at the beginning shortly after.

Try using this language instead:

- Twelve weeks to my first checkpoint in this journey

- I'm two weeks into my journey, long may it continue

- I can't wait for the next challenge after the first twelve weeks of work

Notice I've used words like 'checkpoint', 'journey' and 'next'. This will plant the seed for true transformation, telling your subconscious that there's no end point. Twelve weeks is the starter plan; it's the beginning of your journey towards self-mastery and the body that you've always wanted.

Twelve weeks, or whichever timeframe you determine as your first checkpoint, actually marks the true beginning of your journey. That's where the real hard work starts. Getting into shape is the easy part; learning how to maintain that in your daily life over a long period of time is the hard part. That's what I'm here to address.

WHAT DO I DO NEXT?

A huge problem with any time-sensitive plan or course is the singular focus on the timeframe, which means there's little to no information or guidance on what to do next. You're left in No Man's Land: a dangerous place where you'll see the classic rebounds, binges and lack of control.

What this lack of knowledge of the long-term process has created is the idea that you're either in shape or not. It gives no consideration to staying in shape.

It's time to create a mind shift here. In this book, I'll be taking you step-by-step through the five phases of the transformation journey, including how to walk through the murky waters that come after the first checkpoint – phase three, the consolidation phase – and what to expect.

WHAT AND HOW?

The word 'diet' has a long list of negative connotations. You may associate it with restriction, deprivation and misery. Of course, there is a level of sacrifice you need to make to create a change in your body, but many people believe that health and fitness are neither sustainable nor conducive to maintaining a certain lifestyle (with family, friends, work commitments, etc).

This comes from a lack of education on what we can achieve and how to achieve it. If we can get into shape while still living our favoured lifestyle, we'll believe we can maintain healthy living after our first checkpoint. If we become recluses to get into shape, we're going to lack the self-belief to continue, no matter how good our initial change is.

That's why building long-term lifestyle solutions, understanding meal hygiene and creating a high level of self-awareness become so important. Mastering these different components (which we'll come on to later in the book) trumps the simple act of following a set diet plan.

UNDERPIN IT ALL WITH WHY

CASE STUDY: WHY AM I EVEN DOING THIS?

Let's discuss an example. Two friends, Alice and Sophia,[3] start a transformation together. Alice's reason is purely aesthetically driven, with her only focus being an upcoming holiday to Ibiza in twelve weeks' time. She wants to look good on the beach, fit into a new bikini and take some great holiday snaps.

Sophia's going on the same girls' trip to Ibiza. Her goal is to drop two dress sizes so she'll have the confidence to wear her old clothes again and rock a bikini at the beach parties. She says that when she feels confident, she's bolder at work, takes more ownership of her relationships and has a spring in her step. Sophia's up for promotion in six months' time, and knows that this physical transformation, with the initial Ibiza checkpoint, will be the foundation for her to gain this promotion.

---

3 Names have been changed.

> Both friends have similar initial goals – but look at how differently they've articulated them. Who do you think will succeed most in the short *and* long term? Who is more likely to continue when life gets in the way? Who will push through all challenges, obstacles and barriers?
>
> The clear winner is Sophia. Why? She's laid down the underpinnings of her journey.

Every successful transformation has a why, and more importantly, a strong why behind the why. It's what allows you to think beyond the first checkpoint and focus on creating real, meaningful change. It becomes the anchor to your life and helps you get through the dark days. With a strong underpinning, you'll know the benefits to your life are too important to *not* succeed, both in the short and long term, which is why spending time discovering your why before beginning the transformational journey is so crucial.

TIME FOR A PARADIGM SHIFT

It's time for a new age. A new beginning. A new way of thinking. It all begins with you: your education, your perceptions and your understanding of how to set yourself up for success.

DISCOVERING YOUR TRIGGER

It takes a certain level of introspection to understand the root cause of why you do anything in life. Transforming your body is no different. While, of course, the physical improvement is an added benefit, it's rarely the real reason.

For people like Sophia, making the connection is easy. For others like Alice, it takes more work, but if you look deep enough within your inner core, you'll find it. And it's this discovery you want to connect with, explore and clamp down on. This is critical.

Let's start with your trigger. Before you picked up this book, a switch will have flipped at some point – a trigger to spark a charge. It may have happened in the split second you saw the title, or it may have built up over time, but it's important to recognise what triggered you to pick up this book.

The common initial triggers are:

- Looking back at photos and seeing how far you've slipped

- A passing comment

- Having trouble fitting into clothes

These triggers are like sparks that force action. They're not necessarily the same as your underlying why; in fact, they will typically be more superficial, but they trigger thought and focus your understanding on your true why.

Ask yourself:

- Why have you chosen to learn more about the journey to mastering your body?

- Why are you spending time in your busy day educating yourself on how to be in the shape of your life, for life?

- What problem in your life do you want to solve?

It could be one of many reasons, for example:

- Understanding your mind, body and behaviour to a greater level

- Discovering a unique long-term lifestyle solution that works for you

- Learning how to be in the shape of your life, for life

Now let's ask why you're on this transformation journey. What has your trigger identified the need to do? What's driving you to make a change in your body and life? For example:

- Improve your self-confidence and self-esteem

- Feel, look and perform at your best

- Battle old insecurities, anxiety and/or depression

- Offset future health issues

- Create generational health

- Recover from a bad break-up or loss

- Form an outlet or anchor in the day

- Boost productivity and performance at work

- Inspire your family

- Regain control of your life

Your why will rarely be a physical reason. When you identify the real muck that caused your desire to change, ie your why behind your why, you start to understand that your body is a representation of your mind. Focusing on the physical will be the vehicle to the greater good in your life: the foundation and springboard to propel you forward in all areas. There will be a compounding domino effect across the board, because how you do one thing is how you will do everything.

IDENTIFYING THE MUCK

There will be a specific distress or pain point that you want to get out of. Ask yourself:

- Why have I got here?

- What am I uncomfortable about?

- Who do I want to become?

The work you do to uncover your mindset at the start of this journey underpins everything because the mind and body work together to transform your life. True transformation comes from both, and you need to identify the muck first so you can eliminate it in the phases to come.

Expect to learn some home truths as you understand where you're struggling in your life and what poor lifestyle choices you've been adopting recently to fill the void, find comfort and maybe even seek protection from the outside world. It could be a bad relationship that doesn't serve you; an unful-filling career that causes daily stress; a childhood memory or experience that continues to haunt you, subconsciously or not; even boredom. The reason isn't always obvious, but it's this pain point that forms your why to make a change.

Getting into shape is the tip of the iceberg. It's the vehicle. As you go through the journey, this vehicle will expose the distress to a deeper level and unpack a can of worms. That's why I call it the best self-development tool available.

You need clear underpinnings to your journey because life will always throw challenges at you. Life has a funny way of making things hard when you least expect it, which is when you're most likely to fall off and quit. If you quit at the first hurdle, you'll go nowhere. Your 'why' underpinning every-thing you do will need to be strong enough to keep you on your feet and fighting.

Don't expect an easy ride, because this journey will push you to the limit, physically and mentally. It'll take you to the brink. And that's where you'll find the greatest growth and pleasure. That's where you'll gain the introspection, insights and ideas to unlock a new level of mastery for you. It may happen in the early stages, or it may come later in your journey, but if you stick with it, you will experience this.

I've learnt more about myself trying to master my body than anything else I've done. The journey beyond the first checkpoint is immensely rewarding. Brutally hard, but rewarding. Be excited to lean in.

OVERRIDING THE CHAOS

At the starting blocks of your transformation now, you're likely to be feeling overwhelmed. You may be asking yourself:

- How do I even start?

- How can I change what I've spent five, ten, twenty years doing?

- How do I fit any of this around my busy lifestyle?

This is normal. The good news is you've taken the hardest step. In reading this book, you've sent a message to your brain that you're on a path of change, discovery and improvement. The how will come. That's the easy bit. That's what the book will teach you.

You're now on the right path.

THE POWER OF JOURNALING

It's time to get introspective. I'd recommend you keep a journal for the exercises and tasks you'll work through in this book and let it evolve into your ultimate self-awareness developer. By observing your thoughts and feelings through journaling, you'll be able to make sense of all the questions that your journey will bring with it. You'll gain a better understanding of yourself. And as you go in search of your aha moment, you'll find reasons for your previous failures and more keys to your future success.

How you journal will be individual to you. I like to spend five to twenty minutes when I wake up, before I start any work, on one of these topics:

- Observing lingering and present thoughts

- Writing out my gratitude and appreciation

- Finding solutions to a problem

- Documenting the dream I woke up from

- Reflecting on recent wins

- Answering the questions I'll ask in the book

You'll find your own style as you build momentum with journaling and explore the best way for this friend to serve you in your quest for self-mastery.

To receive the greatest return on investment, please take the time to do every exercise in this book. Don't come back to it later. Each exercise is strategically ordered, and they all feed into maximising your experience of the journey.

These exercises will plant the seeds for greater introspection in the phases of the transformation journey to come. They'll help you see why it's so important you come out of the chaos and regain control of your life. Your journaling work will allow you to marry a short-term transformation with a long-term lifestyle solution, enabling you to deal with everything in your head, reshape your identity and align your behavioural systems.

Exercise: The Why Behind the Why

This exercise may be easy for you, or it may force you to think hard about why you do what you do, and what's important to you. Turn your wi-fi off, put your phone away, and spend at least thirty minutes answering:

- Why is achieving [goal] important to you?

- Why is [outcome] important to you?

- Why is [outcome #2] important to you?

- Why is [outcome #3] important to you?

Aim for at least ten connections here. Each connection will bring you closer to your highest priority in life. The more you link your journey to this, the stronger your why will be when life gets in the way.

Here is an email excerpt I send to clients as an example of how to complete this exercise. I wrote this during a maintenance period of my life where there was no tangible goal. Without having a strong why, I would have likely deprioritised myself and fallen out of shape.

- *Why is staying in shape important?*
Being lean and strong is important to me because it makes me feel great and gives me stress-free me time.

- *Why is this important to me?*
It helps me be productive and in flow, and grow the business.

- *Why is this important to me?*
So that I can better serve my clients, my team and my family.

- *Why is this important to me?*
So that my clients achieve better results, my team has a stronger client base to work with, and I can be more present with my family and provide them with security.

And so on...

If I don't train, none of this is possible. I wouldn't be able to perform at a high level. Instead, I'd feel stressed, low on energy and unproductive. When I think I'm 'too busy' to look after myself, I connect to my why behind my why and it always forces me into action.

What's your why, and your why behind your why? Are you doing this for your self-confidence? Is it for your children? Is it to battle your old insecurities? Have a think, because if you connect with this why, it will change everything for you.

Your why behind your why will evolve as you move through your journey, so revisit it on a quarterly basis.

THE FIVE-STEP PROCESS TO REAL GOALS

There's a popular belief that if you want to achieve anything, you need a goal. I'd like to challenge that. I'd argue that this goal-setting obsession is contributing to our quick-fix mentality and the lack of sustainable long-term results.

If we always live by goals, we'll likely fall victim to the yo-yo phenomenon. Creating goals around timeframes and specific outcomes can help get us off the ground. It can plan our initial journey and provide a useful steer in the right direction, but it won't help us past that. Once we achieve our goal, we'll be stuck at what to do next and wonder how we're supposed to keep everything we've worked so hard for with no tangible goal in sight. Old habits start creeping in again, and we're back to square one.

What we need to focus on instead is building our structure, strategy and systems, and falling in love with the journey. That's where the magic lies. The blueprint I'm going to give you will allow you to win for life, and continuously make improvements.

While goals shouldn't be the sole focus, they still hold value at the beginning of your journey. Here's the five-step process I like to use:

1. Discover your why.

2. Explore your why behind your why.

3. Set a long-term goal of who you want to be.

4. Set a realistic short-term goal for your first checkpoint, while mapping the journey thereafter.

5. Reverse engineer and build the structure, strategy and systems that enable you to achieve the first checkpoint and set you up to build on your future success.

Notice how goal setting comes after you find your why. A goal in itself won't lift you up when the chips are down; you need to know why you're on this journey, why it's important to you and who it'll allow you to become. Only after understanding this can you set the short-term checkpoint goals to steer you along the way.

CASE STUDY: PREPARATION FOR A PHOTOSHOOT

Here's an example from my journal. It was June 2019, before starting preparation for a photoshoot in September. Notice how I cover each of the five steps.

'I'll always train, eat well and look after my health and wellbeing. It's the anchor in my day. It brings me structure, activates a meditative state that keeps me sane, and allows me to perform at my best at all times. More recently, I've let my rules slip a little, and I don't enjoy the feeling. I still look good and maintain solid shape year-round, but I'm more lethargic and less productive. I'm making poor decisions, my stress levels are high, and I'm anxious a lot of the time.

'I need to sharpen the sword. I need to practise what I preach. I need to prioritise myself again and remember that if I want to take care of everyone around me, I have to take care of myself first. I need an upgrade.

'That's my why, and my why behind my why. If I want to build RNT, I have to lead from the front and be at my best at all times. I can't do that if I'm feeling like this. If I want to be better in my relationships with my family and friends, I have to be at my best. I need a reset to realign myself and adapt my lifestyle solution to how I live and operate now.

'To get the wheels in motion for the next part of this journey and create a short-term focus, I've booked a photoshoot in twelve weeks. I know the best way to bring the focus back is to get into extreme condition, so it's the perfect checkpoint. After this, I'll focus on consolidating my results, before investing in myself through the next phase to allow continuous improvement in my day-to-day habits and routines to maintain the new upgrade. To start with, I need to audit what I'm doing now, book the photoshoot for extra accountability, and consult with my coach on how to build the initial structure, strategy and systems that'll lead to my long-term success.'

A day later...

'I know what I need to do now based on what's been going wrong recently. Instead of training three to four days a week, I'm going to push it to five to six, and I'll train on a high-intensity, low-volume approach, which I love. This will give me the weekly structure I crave as I work from home. I'll eat 1,800 calories split into three meals, prepped two days at a time, and eaten at 11am, 3pm and 7pm.'

The journal entry continues to discuss the instructions from my coach, and the daily processes required to reach my new identity and transformation goals, both in the short and long term.

CREATING REALISTIC EXPECTATIONS

What I've noticed over the years is that we all tend to have attachments to certain numbers on the scale. For men, it's typically 60 kg, 65 kg, 70 kg, 75 kg or 80 kg. For women, it's typically 45 kg, 50 kg, 55 kg or 60 kg.

While the scale is not the be-all and end-all, it does provide an objective data point to measure progress. The problem is in expectations and the misconceptions the media have created. It's funny how often I hear:

- I want to be 80 kg 'shredded'

- I only need to drop about 5 kg

- I don't want to go below [insert number] bodyweight

These goals are normally far-fetched and unrealistic, but I don't blame people when I consider the focus of the mainstream and social media. All we get from it is frustration, stress and living in search of the magic bullet.

I was exactly the same for years. In 2014, before my first bodybuilding show, I remember asking my coach:

'How much weight do you think I need to lose, and what bodyweight will I end up at?'

I thought I knew the answer already. I was 84 kg, as strong as I'd ever been, and thought I'd need to lose about 8 kg to be ready. His answer completely threw me.

'You need to lose about 13 to 15 kg and will likely end up around 70 kg.'

He wasn't wrong. Seventeen weeks later and I was ready at exactly 70 kg.

This was my first taste of the reality of natural physique development. In 2017, it was the same story. I reached a bodyweight best of 90 kg in my muscle-building phase, only to need twenty-one weeks to lose 18.5 kg to end up at 71.5 kg (considered a middleweight in the competition I entered). I was far more muscular and conditioned than I'd been in 2014, but I was still nowhere near the numbers that I thought I'd be when I started training ten years prior.

The good news is that over the years, I've been able to spot the trends. The consensus is:

Most people overestimate how much muscle they have, and underestimate how much body fat they carry.

This belief is what creates the attachment and fear to go below the scale numbers.

When setting your first checkpoint goal, you need realistic lean bodyweight (BW) targets. Here are the targets for the everyday person with average levels of muscle mass and genetics.[4]

---

4   In this example, being lean refers to clear definition of abdominals (ie a six pack) at your transformation checkpoint, if that's your goal. This may not be the same as the bodyweight you aim to maintain in the long term (which will depend on your strategy in phases four and five).

Male		Female	
Height (metres)	**BW target (kg)**	**Height (metres)**	**BW target (kg)**
1.62–1.69	54–63	1.52–1.57	40–48
1.7–1.76	58–68	1.58–1.65	44–52
1.77–1.80	63–75	1.66–1.73	48–56
1.81+	68–80	1.74–1.77	52–60

There will be overlap here, and I have generalised, but these numbers fall in line with the data my team and I at RNT have collected over the years. The factors to consider when thinking about where you'll fall on the range are:

- Training experience

- Levels of muscle mass

- Genetics

If you're someone with a few years of training experience, a good level of muscle tissue and average genetics, then there's a 99% chance you'll fall into these parameters. For those of you in the first two years of training, expect to be on the lower end. Unless you're blessed with incredible genetics, it's going to take time to build muscle, which is why once you complete your fat-loss phase and reach your first checkpoint, what comes after is so important.

If you see a picture of someone and wonder why you don't look like them despite being a similar height, it's likely they've been training more consistently for longer, and they've spent more time in phases focused on improving their bodies.

Your goal shouldn't be to compare yourself, but to continue improving yourself.

CASE STUDY: SHYAM

Shyam's the perfect example here. As a city executive who'd let the London culture of eating out and drinking cause him to slip up on his habits, he shared his progress up to his first checkpoint on the internet and it went viral.

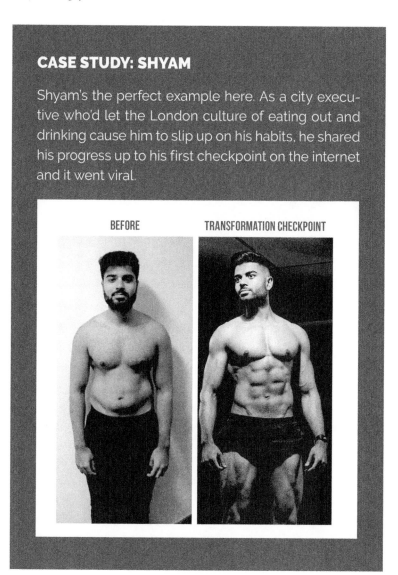

BEFORE

TRANSFORMATION CHECKPOINT

Impressive, right?

Shyam's on the high end of the ranges listed (63 kg at 1.69 m). The reason for this is that, despite having spent years yo-yoing without a long-term lifestyle solution, he had spent a long time training and building up a base. By the time he put his effort into working through the five phases, he was able to display an incredible physique at his first transformation checkpoint, the point at which he was in the shape of his life.

To read the week-by-week journey to Shyam's first transformation checkpoint, go to www.rntfitness. com/book-bonuses.

Understanding realistic expectations isn't meant to discourage you or set limiting beliefs. It's to save you from the frustration, stress and disappointment I and so many others have been through. I was once told I needed to be 85 kg and super lean to set a good example to my clients on the gym floor. At the time, I was 78–79 kg in OK condition, so I had about 10 kg of muscle to gain to be able to meet that objective.

I didn't know better. I thought I could achieve this. But I kept banging my head against a brick wall. The reality was I was never going to achieve this goal without a new set of genetics or using performance-enhancing drugs. Once I accepted that I was never going to be 85 kg super lean, it freed me to stop stressing out, removed the comparison syndrome and allowed me to focus on running my own race.

By taking the time to understand what's realistic, you embrace your own journey, enjoy the benefits and set better short- and long-term goals for what you want to achieve and who you want to become.

CASE STUDY: MANEET

It was the time of the week for Maneet, a private sedation dentist in his thirties from Los Angeles, to check in. He had a photoshoot coming up and was sitting around the 66 kg mark. Having started his journey at 84 kg, he was doing well, but if he wanted to achieve photoshoot condition at his first checkpoint, he needed to drop another 4–5 kg.

As I opened the email, I had a sense of what Maneet was about to report. I'd been there countless times before. Here was the main point:

'I've dropped shy of a kilo this week and I'm now 66 kg. I think this is a good place; from the start, I said I was aiming for 70 kg, and I didn't have any plans to get below that. I'm now at 66 kg. While I'm looking good, I don't want to go below 65 kg, let alone reach the 60 kg target you have in mind for this photoshoot.'

Once we realigned with how he wanted to look at his first checkpoint, he understood that he needed to continue dropping. On the day of his photoshoot, he weighed in at just above 60 kg. He was in the shape of his life with the physique he'd always envisioned. He'd reached his transformation checkpoint, and it was time to transition to the next phase.

In an exchange almost a year later, Maneet wrote:

'I had no idea what it took to get into shape. I had many mental blocks at each mini checkpoint I reached, and when I was at the 65 kg mark, I almost settled for less than my best. I'm so glad I didn't. The next 5 kg changed my life. It shaped the success and results generated in the next phases. I was able to learn how hard I could push my body, and then take that knowledge to consolidate and build my lifestyle solution. I now stay within a few kilos of my lowest weight year-round. I love it.'

🌐 To learn how Maneet built a lifestyle solution to drop nearly 25 kg and transform his life, go to www.rntfitness.com/book-bonuses.

Exercise: Reverse engineer your start

Now you know where you're heading to for your first checkpoint, it's time to reverse engineer where you want to be to where you are now.

If you use the general rule of losing 1% bodyweight per week, this will give you an approximate length of time to reach your first checkpoint. Even if your short- and long-term goal is muscle building, you may want a 'priming' phase to set yourself up for future success. Getting leaner and working towards the realistic body-weight ranges will allow you to maximise the process afterwards.

There are other factors to consider here, though. It's not always as simple as losing 1% bodyweight per week. It depends on:

- Your initial body fat levels

- The amount of time you have to train and be active

- How much your time structure and non-negotiables are set towards your fat-loss goal

- If you've successfully dieted and/or achieved the physique you're after previously

These factors, combined with knowing what you'll weigh when you're lean, will allow you to set a realistic timeframe for your first checkpoint. You have to be honest with yourself here, connect to your why and objectively consider your commitment to change.

If after working this out, you feel discouraged because you won't reach your first checkpoint for at least fifty weeks, understand that it doesn't matter. My favourite analogy is if it's taken you twelve years to walk into the woods, you can't expect to walk back out in twelve weeks. You're on your own path. Work through the phases in your own time, while not distracting yourself with any comparison syndrome. This is what will lead to long-term sustainability and true transformation.

Creating a timeframe is important as without a deadline, you procrastinate. If you procrastinate, you won't apply the internal focus required to reap all the benefits of this journey. A deadline is one part of the equation in facilitating massive action. Accountability is the second.

THE POWER OF ACCOUNTABILITY

By working through the exercises in this chapter so far, you are likely to have created a strong sense of personal commitment and self-accountability. Self-accountability is critical to any transformation journey. It forces excellence in your actions, holds you to high standards, and builds self-esteem as you tick the boxes required to achieve the desired outcomes.

It doesn't stop there, though. Relying only on self-accountability will backfire, especially when things get tough. Then self-doubt, self-sabotage and procrastination can set in – even if you have a checkpoint deadline in place. You need to add another layer of accountability: peer accountability.

Tell everyone around you what you're doing. You may cringe when you see a friend post up their progress on social media, but what they're doing is adding layers to their accountability systems. When you tell your family, friends and colleagues what you're doing, why it's important to you, and what you want to achieve from it, they'll hold you accountable and support you. While this journey is your own, it's not easy alone. Having a strong support system and peer-level accountability can make it more enjoyable, fruitful and successful.

It doesn't stop there, either. There's one more layer that has the power to amplify everything – a professional coach who has a proven track record in helping people with similar goals to yours, and who practises what they preach. Leonardo DiCaprio, Serena Williams, Bill Clinton and Oprah Winfrey, to name but a few successful people, have all had a mentor to learn from and hold themselves accountable to.

A good coach or mentor can show you the blueprint to your individual success and hold you accountable to taking action and making progress every day. You'll learn the tools, strategies and solutions to the predictable mistakes, challenges and obstacles everyone faces on the journey, and you'll save invaluable time and money in the process.

There's no original problem. An experienced results-producing professional coach can provide the insight you need to master your journey and fulfil your potential.

Exercise: What are your accountability systems?

Think about the support system around you, and ask yourself:

- Which family members, friends and peers will you tell your goals and your why to?

- Is there an accountability group you can form with your peers?

- Is there an existing group of like-minded people all striving towards similar goals that you can join?

Exercise: Pause and revise

Now that you've rewired your outlook to the journey ahead, it's time to pause for a moment. I want you to re-read all your notes on:

- Your why

- Your why behind your why

- Your goal

- Your first checkpoint timeframe

- Your accountability systems

Keep these in mind as we work through the five-phase methodology to being in the shape of your life, for life. It's time for a new beginning. When you're ready, let's dive in.

THE FIVE PHASES OF YOUR TRANSFORMATION JOURNEY

One of the biggest lessons I've learnt since I started coaching clients in 2010 is that in a productive and successful transformation journey, there's no on or off switch. It's a lifestyle that evolves through different phases that all interlink and feed off each other to create a unique system, enabling us to transform in the best possible way. Each phase serves its own purpose. Those who go through all the phases not only get into the shape of their lives, but stay there and continue to improve.

Having built a global coaching team to work with thousands of busy people, I've realised how predictable this journey is. It's unique and personal in how it unravels, but it's predictable in the outcomes, strategies and challenges it presents at different stages.

Here are the phases of the RNT Transformation Journey:

PHASE ONE – CLEAN THE PALATE

This is where you regain control of your day, build positive habits, and create a structure, strategy and system that works for you. A well-executed clean the palate (CTP) phase will build the foundation for future success. Get it wrong, and you'll be stuck here forever; spinning your wheels in the search for something that works.

PHASE TWO – PROCESS

After forming your unique structure, strategy and system during CTP, you build momentum and start pushing hard towards your initial goal. If you're successful here, you'll reach your transformation checkpoint and be in the shape of your life. Failure here can be for many reasons, from a lack of lifestyle solutions and poor underpinnings to the journey, to low levels of accountability.

PHASE THREE – CONSOLIDATION

This is the critical period of maintaining what you've achieved so far where you need to change your thinking and perceptions, and fight internal battles against losing the control you have. The majority fail at this point, which is why so many people are able to get into shape, but very few can keep it up. The dieting industry relies on the failure of this stage.

PHASE FOUR – INVESTMENT

If you successfully consolidate, you're in the position to test yourself in a new capacity. You start working on creating further physique improvements while refining your lifestyle solutions. This is a lengthy phase. It requires patience, short and long-term goal setting, and a shift in behaviour, mindset and identity to continue building on the productive work so far.

PHASE FIVE – REWARD

The holy grail. Your mind, body and life are unre-cognisable as you enjoy being in the shape of your life, for life. You don't settle here, though, as you continue to seek improvement and strive for higher levels of self-mastery through new challenges. Few will reach this point. It takes years of hard work but is worth it for the life-changing benefits.

PHASE 1 - CLEAN THE PALATE

- (RNT) REGAIN CONTROL OF YOUR DAY AND BUILD HABITS
- ✓ CREATE A STRATEGY, SYSTEM AND STRUCTURE THAT WORKS FOR YOU
- ? 'HOW DO I DO THIS?'

PHASE 2 - THE PROCESS

- (RNT) PUSH HARD TOWARDS YOUR INITIAL FAT LOSS GOALS
- ✓ ACHIEVE FIRST TRANSFORMATION CHECKPOINT
- ? 'HOW HARD CAN I PUSH MYSELF?'

PHASE 3 - CONSOLIDATION

- (RNT) THE CRITICAL PERIOD OF MAINTAINING WHAT YOU'VE ACHIEVED
- ✓ DEVELOP INSIGHTS ON YOURSELF AND YOUR LIKES/DISLIKES
- ? 'HOW DO I KEEP WHAT I'VE BUILT?'

PHASE 4 - INVESTMENT

- (RNT) IMPROVE YOUR PHYSIQUE FURTHER AND CREATE LIFESTYLE SOLUTIONS
- ✓ TEST YOURSELF IN A NEW CAPACITY
- ? 'HOW DO I BUILD ON THIS?'

PHASE 5 - REWARD

- (RNT) TIME TO ENJOY BEING IN THE SHAPE OF YOUR LIFE, FOR LIFE
- ✓ CONTINUOUS IMPROVEMENT AND SELF MASTERY
- ? 'HOW CAN I KEEP GETTING BETTER?'

Knowing these predictable phases guides you through your journey, allowing you to see what's next and build your confidence that there's a solution to every problem you'll encounter. Most people I speak to have never experienced what comes after the first transformation checkpoint, and that comes back to the purpose of this book. That's my why.

The five phases are the same for everyone. They will happen in the same order, regardless of your background and history. It's easy to believe that your situation is different and that it's not possible to stay in shape with your lifestyle, or that you can skip phases. My team and I have worked with every background, story, struggle you could put forward. In reality, the only difference between people will be the amount of time they spend in each phase.

I liken the five phases to building a brand-new customised house from the ground up. There are specific stages to follow, rules to abide by and ways to accelerate progress, and they're all in place to allow us to design a house that we love that works for us in the long run. While the approach is unique, the trajectory of the journey always follows the same predictable path.

By the end of this book, you'll know how to navigate through each of the five phases. You'll have the tools to finally get into the shape of your life, for life. Follow the path and you'll experience all the incredible benefits that transcend the physical: improved self-confidence, better relationships, a more productive career and a new-found zest for life.

For now, have a think about where you may have failed in the past, and which phase you've always struggled to go through. As we work through the phase you're thinking about, keep an eye out for your aha moment. You'll know when it strikes.

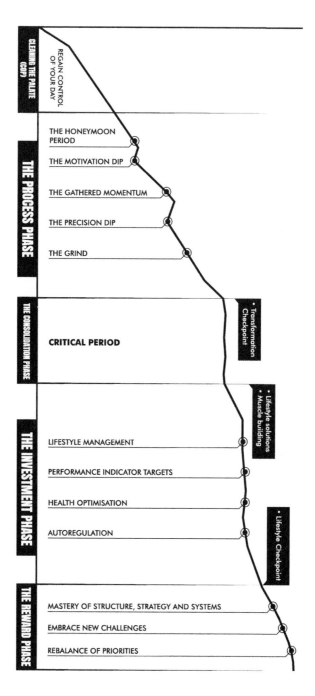

HOW TO GET INTO THE SHAPE OF YOUR LIFE, FOR LIFE

CLEANING THE PALATE (CBP)

REGAIN CONTROL OF YOUR DAY

THE PROCESS PHASE

THE HONEYMOON PERIOD

THE MOTIVATION DIP

THE GATHERED MOMENTUM

THE PRECISION DIP

THE GRIND

THE CONSOLIDATION PHASE

CRITICAL PERIOD

• Transformation Checkpoint

THE INVESTMENT PHASE

• Lifestyle solutions
• Muscle building

LIFESTYLE MANAGEMENT

PERFORMANCE INDICATOR TARGETS

HEALTH OPTIMISATION

AUTOREGULATION

• Lifestyle Checkpoint

THE REWARD PHASE

MASTERY OF STRUCTURE, STRATEGY AND SYSTEMS

EMBRACE NEW CHALLENGES

REBALANCE OF PRIORITIES

YOUR JOURNEY IS YOUR OWN

The growth of social media and ease of information access means comparison syndrome is at an all-time high. It's near impossible to escape if you're not careful. But while the journey is predictable from a big-picture macro level, the micro nuances are individual to you.

Ultimately, your journey is your own. No one has a better journey, only different. Approaching each phase with this understanding can alleviate any debilitating stress from unnecessary comparisons with others that may slow down your progress. Any stories, timeframes or strategies I use as case studies are individual to the people involved. Your situation is likely to be different, so approach this book with the macro in mind, and then figure out how the micro applies to you.

IT'S NEVER JUST ABOUT THE PHYSICAL

When I first started my career in 2010, I thought I was entering the field of personal training with a focus on body transformation. As I worked with more clients over the years, I realised I wasn't only changing bodies, I was changing lives. The penny dropped shortly after I launched RNT in 2017, when I began to receive scores of emails from people around the world who were raving about the benefits they were experiencing from their transformation journeys.

What was interesting was their feedback rarely mentioned their physical changes. It was everything but: their mental health, mindset, careers, relationships all improved. The physical process of transforming the body provided the vehicle they needed to make the necessary changes in other areas of life.

I've experienced this in myself over the past decade. I was the 'skinny fat' seventeen-year-old with moobs and a pot belly who would constantly seek approval, lacked self-confidence and had low self-esteem. The physical was the vehicle for me to change my life for the better, and it still is. Even over a decade later, taking care of my physical being is the anchor to my day. It's a focus. It's all encompassing. Any time I let my daily rules, structure, strategy and systems slip, everything else in my life falls apart.

Being in the shape of your life, for life is about taking care of the number-one person in your life – you. If you can master your physical being, you'll have the confidence and courage to master any domain in your life. You'll have the inward focus and the positive structures, strategies and systems in place to push forward in any area you want to improve. It's the ultimate teacher and vehicle to set yourself up for success.

Life is never the same once you've gone through the transformational journey. It teaches you to think critically, analyse situations and work out solutions. It enables you to handle whatever life throws at you. The bonus? You'll be in the shape of your life, for life.

2
PHASE ONE: CLEANING THE PALATE

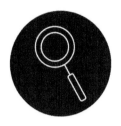

The aim of CTP is to regain control of your day, build habits, and create a structure, strategy and system that work for your unique lifestyle in the long term. Every transformation journey begins with phase one, CTP. It's the foundation phase where you lay down the bricks to facilitate long-term lifestyle solutions.

You're likely to experience fast results in the short and medium term as you regain control and make significant changes to your day to day. You'll create the anchor for your journey as you rigorously audit yourself while figuring out what works for your lifestyle. When you're coming out of chaos in a state of overwhelm, doubt and fear, knowing your why, your why behind your why, your goal and your accountability system will make laying down the foundation much easier.

This time you're not just 'starting a diet'; you're thinking beyond the first checkpoint. You're building your unique long-term lifestyle solution to be in the shape of your life, for life, and enjoy all the benefits this brings. You're going against the grain here, which can be uncomfortable. That's OK.

The first step of CTP is to master the 3Ss:

- Structure

- Systems

- Strategy

The 3Ss, in combination with the CTP accelerators, which we'll come on to later in this chapter, are the priority for this phase. Typically, CTP will last between fourteen and twenty-eight days, depending on individual context and circumstances. It may even be more; I've seen people spend up to six months in a CTP phase because they needed more time to refine their initial 3Ss before making the push the next phase requires. The time frame is irrelevant; if you enter the next phase without mastering your 3Ss, you'll quickly go back to square one.

Real habits that require no thinking to execute take a long time to form. A 2009 study found it can take anywhere from 18 to 254 days, depending on the individual, difficulty and various other factors.[4] But a process that you repeat that's high on your priority list will get easier every day. Think tiny steps. Create small wins and build-up momentum one day at a time.

---

4 Lally, P; van Jaarsveld, C H M; Potts, H W W; Wardle, J (2010) 'How Are Habits Formed: Modelling habit formation in the real world'. *European Journal of Social Psychology.*

MASTERING THE 3Ss

Transforming your body will require you to perform specific actions on a daily basis that on the surface look simple. These actions make up your transformation checklist.

RNT TRANSFORMATION CHECKLIST:

- ✔ Strength train three to four days per week
- ✔ Follow your nutrition plan, staying within a calorie deficit (if after fat loss)
- ✔ Drink 3–4 litres of water a day
- ✔ Take at least 10,000 steps a day
- ✔ Sleep seven to eight hours a night

The actions for each person will vary, but the general guidelines will stay true for anyone striving to reach their first checkpoint. There are thousands of books and plans out there which will tell you how to train, eat and be healthy. What's missing is how you execute this in the real world with family, work, socials and life to contend with.

Enter the 3Ss.

STRUCTURE

Structure equals freedom. As counterintuitive as it may sound, if you want to have the freedom to control what's happening in your day, you need excellent structure. If you're going into your days winging it, expect to fail miserably. CTP all starts with finding a structure that works for you. Everyone is different.

Would you want to build a house on top of weak foundations? I'd put money on the house falling down if you did. If you have no structure, no discipline, no rules, are you truly free? You might feel like it for a second, but absolute freedom is a paradox. The problem with living a life of absolute freedom is you'll always be a second away from collapse. Your house won't be able to withstand a storm, and by default, you'll be unable to overcome the overwhelm you're likely to feel at the start of a transformation journey.

Novelist Paulo Coelho famously said, 'Discipline and freedom are not mutually exclusive, but mutually dependent, because without discipline we would sink into chaos.'[5] I consider discipline to be an outcome of having a solid structure so, bearing in mind Coelho's quote, having more structure will breed more freedom. It allows you to get the things, feelings and actions you want from your day. It'll enable you to weather more storms in your life without constantly dealing with the aftermath. And it'll give you the chance to focus on what truly matters, work on the muck you've identified and execute accordingly.

To help create better structure, you need to instil rules. Having rules will allow you to build a better house and enable you to incorporate the other two S's – system and strategy – into

---

5 Coelho, P (2017) 'Discipline and freedom are not mutually exclusive' [Facebook post] 23 February 2017. www.facebook.com/paulocoelho/photo s/a.241365541210/10154880056531211/?type=1&theater

your life more efficiently. The rules that may be pertinent for your lifestyle solution could include:

- **Waking up earlier.** By adding more time to your day, you automatically give yourself a head start and feel less overwhelmed.

- **Planning your days and weeks in advance.** You may not be able to predict everything that will happen, but planning 60–70% of your day and week will give you the freedom to be present in the moment, productive and in control.

- **Creating themes for parts of your day.** For example, my themes for the day are as follows: mornings are for myself (train, write and walk); afternoons are for work (emails, projects, meetings); and evenings are for loved ones (family and friends).

Rules are individual, yet essential. In a world of chaos and overwhelm, having rules, structure and discipline can help you make sense of life. They give you the framework to build your transformation journey around. I'm not implying you can't have any flexibility in your life at all; being adaptable to different situations is important, but being adaptable in the face of no ground rules can make life difficult.

Exercise: Formulating your structure

- How can you create more structure in your day according to your why, your priorities and your goals?

- Can you create themes for your day?

SYSTEMS

Systems are everything. If you want to get your foot off the ground with your transformation, you need systems. These are the surface-level requirements of getting into the best shape possible. If you reverse engineer your first checkpoint, your system to achieve the goal is to tick the five boxes of the transformation checklist on a daily and weekly basis, but we need to take it a step further and discuss how you will do this. We need a system for the system.

Exercise: Building your systems

What is your system for:

- Training three to four days a week?

- Following your nutrition plan every day?

- Drinking 3–4 litres of water a day?

- Taking 10,000 steps a day?

- Sleeping seven to eight hours a night?

Focusing on the goal of accomplishing these can be daunting and overwhelming. Creating a system for each is where success lies. Your goal during CTP is to design your system for accomplishing the processes required to achieve your long-term goal.

Let's now break down the transformation checklist further. Ask yourself these questions, keeping in mind your lifestyle requirements and overall structure for the week.

Training:

- Which days of the week will you train?

- What times of the day will you train?

- Where will you train?

Nutrition:

- How many meals a day will you eat?

- When will you prepare your meals for the day/week?

- What times of the day will you eat?

Water intake:

- How will you track your water intake?

- Which water bottle will you carry with you?

- Where will you keep your water bottle?

Steps:

- Where can you add more steps into your day?

- What times of the day are you active and sedentary?

- How can you multitask to save time while accumulating steps?

Sleep:

- What time will you sleep?

- What time will you wake up?

- What will you avoid doing that would affect your sleep?

> By breaking your systems down, you can start putting the pieces of the puzzle together. Through creating systems, you will by default add more structure into your day. As a result, you'll be less overwhelmed and more in control of your life.
>
> Don't overlook the importance of this step. Take your journal out and ask yourself these questions to gain more clarity on the path that lies ahead.

STRATEGY

Strategy is your navigator for when life happens. You've built a structure, you've created your systems, and now you need a strategy to manoeuvre around the challenges of the modern-day lifestyle. Luckily, with the right framework for your day in place, you'll have the rules and form habits that will allow you to execute on your strategy effectively.

Strategy is the art of utilising long-term lifestyle solutions. It's understanding how to work around family commitments, social occasions, work events and relationships while still striving towards your goal. A 'lack of time' and being 'too busy' are the two most common excuses I hear from frustrated people who've yet to transform. They'll tell me how they're too 'involved with family', 'slammed at work', or have 'too many socials on' to succeed at their goals. These are the typical Monday to Thursday dieters who spin their wheels by abandoning all structure and systems on the weekends.

What this comes down to is a lack of strategy. Transformation *can* occur while you're still living your life. The answer lies in strategy.

Exercise: Building your strategy

Just like we broke down the systems into chunks, let's do the same with the potential obstacles, barriers and challenging situations you might find yourself in.

Here are a few that could spell disaster:

- A night out with friends

- Kids' day out

- Friday night takeaway with your partner

- Networking event

- Trip away

Life will always get in the way. You can't wait for a clear spell of three years to begin your transformation journey. That's neither realistic nor sustainable. If you want to get into the shape of your life, for life, you need to become a master of strategy.

The first step before executing any strategy is to recon-nect with your why, your why behind your why, and your accountability systems. This will place you in an optimal state to focus on what you need to do.

Let's break the examples down further.

A night out with friends

- Are you going to drink? If so, what are your rules?

- Is there food involved? If so, what will you eat?

- Does the event need to be food or drink focused?

Kids' day out:

- How can you make the day out more active, and involve the whole family?

- What healthy food can you prep for the day that everyone can eat and enjoy?

Friday night takeaway with your partner:

- Do you need to have a takeaway, or can you cook in?

- What choices align both of your tastes and likes?

Networking event:

- Will you eat or drink at the event? If so, what are your rules?

Trip away:

- What are your rules for food and drink when away?

- How will you continue to train and stay active when away?

Exercise: Identifying your cascading trigger and super rule

There is one recurring question to ask yourself:

What is one trigger you need to avoid that will cascade into further bad decisions?

Everyone has a trigger in their daily life that can lead to other poor decisions and, in many cases, abandoning the 3Ss. It could be as simple as when you pick up your phone, where you sit when you're eating, or whether you hit snooze in the mornings. It could be nibbling on the bread basket, having one glass of wine, or going to dinner with a friend who likes a 'blow out'. When devising your 3Ss, you need to be mindful of what rule you can set in stone that kills a thousand other possibilities.

An example I like to refer to is the gluten-free preference that many feel to be the cause of their weight loss and improved wellbeing. The reality is that by eliminating gluten, they've ensured many food choices are now no longer available to them. They face less temptation when out, have reduced options, so eat fewer calories. A gluten-free diet removes potential triggers for many.

Ask yourself:

- What is the one trigger you need to avoid when out and about as you know it will lead to further bad decisions?

- Which people and environments trigger you to abandon your rules?

- Which foods, activities or behaviours form a gateway to other bad behaviours?

- What is one rule you can create for yourself that will help remove many other decisions or potential disasters in your day?

The more specific you can be here, the better.

A rule I have for myself that makes a tremendous difference to how I feel, think and perform is that I don't look at my phone before 11am in the morning, whichever time zone or environment I may be in. Instead, I'll do creative work on the business, train and make a dent in my daily step target. This has become a hard and fast rule that ensures I don't react to the world in the morning; I stay in control of my day and maintain my 3Ss. As a result, my ability to execute on my transformation checklist remains high. If I break this rule, I'm distracted when I train, more inclined to snack throughout the day and waste time I'd otherwise spend working and being active.

Exercise: Uncovering your emotional triggers

Cascading triggers don't only relate to events, locations, environments and the people you're with. Specific times in your week/month/year and/or your emotional state are also at play here.

Examples may include:

- Eating when you're bored and/or feeling low

- Watching TV versus going for a walk when you're stressed and exhausted from work

- Adopting poor lifestyle practices around times of the year that bring up bad memories

These triggers are harder to define and need more self-awareness, but noticing them can be life changing. It enables you to deal with many of the root causes that may be holding you back. By being aware of your emotional triggers, writing them down and working through them, you can rewire your belief system to eliminate poor decisions in your day.

Ask yourself:

- What specific emotional states trigger you to adopt destructive behaviours?

- Where are you using bad lifestyle choices to provide a coping mechanism, fill a void or provide a solution to an underlying problem (the muck)?

- Is the bad lifestyle choice still the solution to the problem, or do you need to rewire the association here?

CASE STUDY: A CRY FOR HELP

It was Christmas Eve when I received an email from Sanjeeta titled 'Help'. At rock bottom, feeling like there was no way out, she needed to use the physical as the vehicle to pull herself out.

This is what she wrote after having done just that:

'Sometimes help finds its way to you in the most unexpected ways. I found this journey at my absolute lowest. I'd gone to my GP a week before Christmas to tell her I couldn't cope with life anymore.

'She told me, "You can't control what other people say to you or how they treat you, but you do have control over how that impacts you and makes you feel."

'The key word that kept running in my head was control. I had no control in my life. I was overwhelmed, my life was in chaos and I was at the bottom of a rabbit hole, desperately trying to crawl out. Life felt unmanageable.

'After the GP appointment, I was listening to Sad FM on repeat when all of a sudden, I heard an RNT transformation story about how a woman just like me – a full-time working mum – used the physical as a vehicle to transform her life.

'I started the journey with phase one, CTP. This changed my life almost immediately. I'd yo-yo dieted, binged and tried everything in the past. But what I'd never done is to ask myself the hard questions, create structure in my day and bring the focus on to myself for once. I spent this time building systems to work around my kids, my working hours and my socials. I created a strategy for every situation and potential obstacle, and I finally had a structure that unlocked freedom in my head. There was light at the top of the rabbit hole now, and I felt ready after CTP to crawl out and proceed on to the next phases.'

Sanjeeta's story isn't uncommon. Her successful CTP phase meant she was able to lay the foundations to fight off her demons, lose 20% of her bodyweight and build a lifestyle solution to stay in shape year-round.

🌐 To read the full account of Sanjeeta's story, go to www.rntfitness.com/book-bonuses.

CTP ACCELERATORS

Formulating your 3Ss can be a difficult task at the start, which is why you need to harness the power of CTP accelerators:

- Managing decision fatigue

- Installing non-negotiables

- Mastering precursors

Let's take a closer look at each.

MANAGING DECISION FATIGUE

Back in 2015, I was meeting a friend for coffee for the sixth time in three weeks. As I walked in, the first thing he said to me was, 'What's with the green and red tops? Every time we meet, you wear the green top on Tuesday and red on Thursday.'

A little startled, I replied, 'It's just easier, I didn't even think about it.'

For the next week, I examined my behaviour with clothes and realised that I was instinctively choosing the exact same clothes every week. Tuesday and Thursday were my half days away from personal training, so I had my half-day outfits. The rest of the time I wore the same socks, joggers, underwear, T-shirt and hoody. When I'd go out in the evenings, it was the same pair of trousers with either a white or black T-shirt.

I decided to do some research into this, and googled, 'Why do I wear the same clothes every day?' The results were astounding. It turns out Steve Jobs, Mark Zuckerberg, Barack Obama and many other public figures have similar practices. They eliminate the decision behind their clothing so they can focus their time and energy on their key purpose in life.[6]

This was interesting and made me think about all the unimportant extra decisions we make on a daily basis, especially regarding food and routine.

How many times have you asked yourself:

- Should I eat chicken or beef?

- Should I go to the gym at 9am or 9pm?

- Should I wear black or grey?

- Should I eat dinner at 6pm or 8pm?

- Should I have three meals or four meals today?

And so on. The brain only has a limited amount of cognitive capacity in the day. If you're wasting this on non-creative aspects of your life, such as food, clothing and routine, you're setting yourself up for failure.

The work of social psychologist Roy F Baumeister highlights three key findings:[7]

- We use willpower to do everything: make decisions, focus, be creative, etc.

- We only have a limited amount of daily willpower. If we use too much early on, our decision making becomes skewed and lazy, crippling our performance.

5   Bloem, C (2018) 'Successful People Wear the Same Thing Every Day'. www.inc.com/craig-bloem/this-1-unusual-habit-helped-make-mark-zuckerberg-steve-jobs-dr-dre-successful.html
6   Baumeister, R F; Tierney, J (2012) *Willpower: Why self-control is the secret to success*. Penguin.

- The ability to make the best possible decision will reduce in relation to the number of options we have.

Think about when you're most likely to cheat on your diet, skip a gym session or fall back on a trigger that you know isn't good for you. It's probably after 5pm, right? That's because you've depleted your willpower and cognitive capacity. You've spent all day making decisions and expending mental energy, so your ability to make good quality decisions has diminished. The answer? Simplify and automate.

What if you already know what you're going to eat, wear, drink, do in training every day? Now there's no risk. You've standardised the non-creative components of your day and can save all your thinking for things that do matter. This is where the power of rules comes into play. It's why having rules around your structure, strategy and systems makes implementation so much easier.

Look back to your transformation checklist. Imagine if you could automate 80% of the things on the list, formulating your 3Ss to fulfil them. That's a recipe for success.

I know variety is the spice of life, but variety will hold you back in the beginning. During CTP, you want to make as few choices as possible, allowing for action rather than thought. The art of 'doing' is top priority here. You want something actionable that you can manipulate once you're in the swing of things. Variety comes afterwards, once you've built your foundation. Flirting with too many choices when you're in a state of chaos and overwhelm can be your downfall.

CASE STUDY: ARCHANA'S AHA MOMENT

I was speaking with a client, Archana, about what her aha moment had been in the past eighteen months. She didn't hesitate in her answer.

'As a working mother of two young boys, I know the horrible feeling of living in a constant state of over-whelm. For years, my life felt chaotic as I juggled motherhood, working and socialising. If I pinpoint the one thing that's changed in the past eighteen months, it's been limiting decisions.

'I've become a minimalist and essentialist wrapped up in one. I aim to make every decision either auto-mated or as easy as possible on a daily basis. This includes what I wear, what I eat and my routine. Eradicating decision fatigue has opened up space in my mind I never knew I had. It's made installing the transformation checklist into my life seamless.'

To learn more about Archana's minimalist approach, go to www.rntfitness.com/book-bonuses.

Exercise: What can you automate?

Over the next week, think about all the situations in your life that you make trivial decisions on. Write them down and ask yourself, 'How can I automate this decision?'

The results are likely to amaze you. The more you can put yourself into positions where there's only one option to commit to, the better your results. Take action now. And learn to find even better ways of automating decisions as you go through the process.

Overwhelm is your biggest obstacle at this stage of your journey, and it always surprises me just how much food is the source of this feeling. Structure equals freedom, and by following these basic tips, you'll be free to focus on what matters.

- **Plan the night before.** Plan how, when and what you'll be doing as much as your situation allows it. Don't make these decisions in the morning if you want to save your willpower tank for the day (are you spotting a theme here?).

- **Meal prepping.** There are a million ways to do this. It could be weekly, twice a week, daily, in portions or specific foods only. It doesn't matter – find what works for you and roll with it. If you eat on the go when at work, find one or two go-to places that allow you to stay on autopilot.

- **Make commitments and non-negotiables.** Doing so eliminates trying to decide whether you should do something or not and helps build your framework. And non-negotiables happen to be the next CTP accelerator we'll be discussing.

INSTALLING NON-NEGOTIABLES

If CTP is the foundation for the transformation journey, the non-negotiables are your individual bricks. It's all about elevating the different components of the transformation checklist to become a priority in your day. You have to create commitments with yourself here to remove the choice of execution.

How many non-negotiables you make a priority will be personal and life dependent, but the core priorities are:

- A commitment to training three to four days a week

- A commitment to following your nutrition plan every day

- A commitment to taking at least 10,000 steps a day

- A commitment to drinking 3–4 litres of water a day

- A commitment to sleeping seven to eight hours per night

Above all, you need to make a cornerstone commitment to finding a solution to any perceived problem you may face. This may be a social event, a holiday, long working hours, hunger, demotivation – anything. In 99% of cases, a pre-planned alternative is all you need. Once you have your non-negotiables in place, you will by default build the right structure in your day, focus on your systems and think about the strategies you use.

Your cornerstone commitment is what will drive you forward in the face of potentially falling backwards. You'll force yourself to connect to your why, utilise your accountability systems and pull together your 3Ss to make progress. This builds confidence and momentum, creating a solid foundation for the next phase of your transformation journey.

Exercise: Make your commitments

- What commitments are you making to yourself?

- Have you made a cornerstone commitment?

MASTERING PRECURSORS

Making commitments, eliminating decisions and having your 3Ss in place is one-half of the battle. The other half is what happens just before you execute. It's the decision before the decision, the moment prior to acting. Ultimately, it's the hinging task that your success of execution hangs on.

Every day you'll face precursors, and your ability to do what you need to do relies on how you approach the situation. You might overthink, have an excuse or lose the battle to a shifting priority. Chances are, though, if your ability to execute is compromised, something about your structure, strategy or system has changed.

That's where becoming hyper aware of and mastering your individual precursors is so critical. Just as you want to eliminate the decision of doing, you also want to eliminate the decision that comes before the action. For example, ask yourself:

- How many times have you put on your gym kit in the morning and not trained?

- How many times have you got an entire week's shopping and not cooked your meals at home?

- How many times have you put on your running shoes when you've arrived home from work and not done your cardio?

In each situation, it's the moment just before the action that's critical. The gym kit, the shopping, the running shoes make or break what happens next. If you want to fulfil your commitments, you need to analyse your day for your existing precursors.

They won't be inherently positive. For example, when you're waiting in a queue, that may be a precursor for you to pull your phone out. When Friday night comes around, that may be a precursor for a big meal out with a heavy drinking session after. You see where I'm going with this?

One example I often hear is people finish work having already made the decision not to carry their gym kit with them. Instead, they've said they'll go after having dinner at home. The problem here is they've combined two precursors that'll make it harder to leave the house once they're there – the simple act of getting home and the eating of a meal. Both will trigger relaxing and shutting down for the day – the opposite to the original intention.

By using positive precursors, such as changing into your gym kit before leaving work, you'll guarantee an increased rate and intensity of sessions completed. This will make it harder to fall back on the 'relaxing' precursor of training after dinner.

The key lesson here is to look at the structure of your day and be self-aware enough to know which precursors are serving you, and which are setting you back. The goal is to unlock more mental capacity and remove the 'should I do this now?' battle in your head.

CASE STUDY: UTILISING PRECURSORS TO WRITE THIS BOOK

When writing this book, I used the same methodology as I would when undergoing a body transformation. I started with my why, set my goals and created my accountability systems. I then progressed to CTP where I built my 3Ss through CTP accelerators, before pushing with the word count in the process phase.

To enable this, I had to review my days to set myself up for success. An important part of this was using precursors to make it as easy and automatic as possible.

I normally wake up at 5.30am and I love to write in the first two to three hours of my day. Here's how I reverse engineer the process:

Start of the week:

- Note down key content to be written

The night before:

- Open up on Word with what I plan to write with a few notes

Wake up and go through morning routine:

- Brush teeth

- Put on gym T-shirt, hoody and tracksuit bottoms (precursor for training later in the day)

- Walk downstairs and drink a mix of lemon and sea salt with water

- Walk to the corner sofa with my laptop bag

- Open up bag and pull out journal (on top of my laptop – a precursor to journal)

- Journal for five to twenty minutes

- Open up laptop, and open up iTunes to play Chopin's *Nocturnes, Op. 9: No.1 in B Flat Minor* on repeat (precursor to start writing)

- Start writing

These stacks of habits and precursors are now automatic, and I continue to use them in my writing. There are no 'Should I write in the morning?' thoughts. It's planned in advance (twice), and then executed as per my precursors.

The big three here are the notes written the night before, the opening of the laptop and the music. Without these, my level of resistance increases ten-fold. It sounds simple, but it's so habitual now that writing 1,000 words a day is easy.

Exercise: Finding your precursor domino

Here are the four steps to mastering the precursors in your day.

1. The precursors have to be the easiest part of the process with the least resistance that can be done at any point without thought. Examples include putting on your running shoes, opening a book, opening an app and buying the groceries. In his book *Atomic Habits*,[8] James Clear calls this the 'Two Minute Rule'. He explains that the new habit you're adding needs to be easy, quick, ie executed in under two minutes, and act as a gateway habit to lead you down the more productive path.

2. Creating these precursors at the turning points in your day will change the way you act. Examples of

---

7 Clear, J (2018) *Atomic Habits: An easy and proven way to build good habits and break bad ones.* Random House Business.

turning points include the morning period, lunch-time at work, immediately after work and the one hour pre-bed. Behavioural scientist Dr B J Fogg[9] calls these 'anchors' because they're solid parts of your life with existing behaviours to which you can attach new habits. If you can put precursors in those times for the daily tasks you want to achieve, you will be in a favourable position to execute.

3. If you already have a solid structure, your best solution is to analyse your day and find precursors to certain things you want to change. If every week you have to use a lot of willpower to achieve some-thing, or if there's a moment where you always fall short, start there. For example, a common problem on a Friday night is the question, 'Shall we just get a takeaway and open a bottle of wine?' To add a posi-tive precursor to prevent this, buy foods conducive to your goals on a Thursday.

4. Analyse your current set up and find situations in your day you want to automate, and then put something in place to make that happen before the event. For example, if you want to stop worrying about whether you're going to eat chicken or turkey on a Monday, plan it the week before, or follow a set meal plan. If getting dressed in the morning causes a ton of stress and zaps your energy, create a 'personal uniform'. You want to automate as many

8   Fogg, B J (2019) *Tiny Habits: The small changes that change everything.* Virgin Books.

> of the menial non-creative components of your day as possible so you can save time and energy for what matters most.

DOES CTP EVER END?

The benefits of the transformation journey will always transcend the physical. Through a successful CTP phase, you will notice an increase in self-confidence. For many of you, this will be the first time you've kept promises to yourself and taken control of your life. That breeds confidence. And it's with this you start noticing shifts in your behaviour, mindset and outlook as you await the challenges in the next phase.

CASE STUDY: ROSHNI SETS HERSELF FREE

I recently asked a client, Roshni, a primary school teacher under pressure on a daily basis, how she felt after her CTP phase. Her words summed up the exact experience and feeling I want you to have after this phase:

'I feel great and I'm beaming with energy. More than that, I'm in control. Having a clear structure in my day has been a game changer. I also love that I don't have any decisions to make in the day. I thought I'd hate the idea of being 'samey', but it's freed my mind and I no longer feel trapped by constant overwhelm. CTP has given the reboot to my system that I was craving – a focus in my day – and I'm ready to push on.'

CASE STUDY: AKASH FINDS THE TIME

My namesake and client, Akash, an active father of two and entrepreneur, could play the 'I'm busy' card and neglect himself, but in the near three years I've been working with him, not once have I heard him complain about time. Few people have this quality, so I asked him what the secret was.

'My why, and my why behind my why, is crystal clear. I know who I want to become. What type of father, husband, friend and business owner I want to be. I know how important focusing on my physical self is to everything else I do in life. With limited time, I focus on creating a structure, strategy and system that works for my lifestyle. For me, this means dominating the morning.

'Getting up before my family, often at 4am, allows me time to train, work and complete tasks that may not have got done otherwise. It's my one thing and secret to my success, but I also have a few strategies and systems that cascade into making everything easier. I spend an hour on Sunday prepping my meals. I keep a treadmill in my home office to make steps a no brainer. And I have firm rules for the frequent networking events I attend.

'Furthermore, I block out non-negotiable time in my week for training. I keep my food similar to limit decisions, and because I train in the morning, I keep my gym kit right by my treadmill to make it easy when I wake up. Spending time over the years refining everything CTP first taught me has been a life changer.'

🌐 To learn more about how Akash and Roshni applied the 3Ss to their busy lifestyles, go to www.rntfitness.com/book-bonuses.

It's all too tempting to skip over the CTP phase and jump right into the home straight of your first checkpoint. Avoid this at all costs. You'll only end up spinning your wheels and finding another shiny object to grab hold of. Instead, lean in, embrace the initial discomfort and plant the seeds for the transformation that awaits you.

As you go through this book, you'll notice a CTP reset feature in each of the phases to come. The function of the CTP reset is to go back to basics, sharpen the sword and realign your focus. Life isn't static, and as your goals and lifestyle demand change, your 3Ss will need to evolve with them.

SUMMARY

CTP goal:

- Regain control of your day

CTP essentials:

- Build your 3Ss – structure, strategy and systems

CTP accelerators:

- Managing decision fatigue

- Installing non-negotiables

- Mastering precursors

Now that you've regained control and started building your 3Ss, let's accelerate your progress to the next level.

3
PHASE TWO: PROCESS

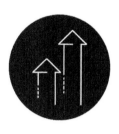

The aim of the process phase is to use everything you've built during CTP to push hard towards your first transformation checkpoint, where you'll complete the first half of the equation: getting into the shape of your life.

TICKING THE BOXES IN FIVE STAGES

The process phase is exactly what it says on the tin. It focuses on the processes – your transformation checklist – required to achieve your first goal. At the same time, it's a teacher, a humbler. It instils patience and consistency while delivering short-term wins along the way.

A productive process phase relies on a successful foundation of CTP, where we worked on:

- Your why, and the why behind your why

- Your goals and expectations

- Your accountability systems

- Your 3Ss (structure, system, strategy)

- Your CTP accelerators (decision fatigue, non-negotiables, precursors)

With your CTP foundations in place, you'll focus on the daily processes versus the checkpoint, which can feel daunting and an impossible feat at this stage. Take it one day, one brick at a time. There's no rush; just like every house build will be different, so will every transformation journey. What took one person sixteen weeks may take you thirty weeks, fifty-two weeks or even longer. That's OK – your journey is your own.

A word of caution: the road to the first checkpoint isn't going to be straightforward, no matter what your timeframe is. There are going to be delays. You're going to encounter problems, obstacles and challenges in every new part of the journey. With these will come distinct feelings that will vary in length, and these feelings make up the five stages of the process phase. They will always happen, but the extent to which they occur and when will be individual to you.

The five stages are:

1. The honeymoon period

2. The motivation dip

3. The gathered momentum period

4. The precision dip

5. The grind

After we've discussed each stage in detail, I'll tell you about the process accelerators you can use to help you navigate through them.

THE HONEYMOON PERIOD

Ah, the fun times. Think about any new project you've started. Once you get past the initial overwhelm of what you need to do, it's great. Progress is fast. It's exciting, fun and you want to go as quickly as you can.

In stage one of the process phase, you're riding the wave of the early momentum you've built up during CTP to rack up some big wins. You're nailing your transformation checklist every day. You're losing 1% of your bodyweight per week at least. Everything is looking rosy, and you'll probably be wondering why you found it so hard the last time you attempted it. How could you have failed in your pursuit of the checkpoint, and more, before? You begin to think bigger; you question whether your goal is hard enough, and you start picturing reaching your first checkpoint a little earlier than expected.

Then stage two hits you...

THE MOTIVATION DIP

Novelty always wears off. What was sexy suddenly feels samey. After four to eight weeks of building consistency on your 3Ss and CTP accelerators, while experiencing some initial changes, you'll encounter what's known as the motivation dip.

Despite nailing all the processes and seeing all the metrics heading in the right direction, you're likely to question why you're now not seeing much physical change. The initial transformation is nowhere near complete, and you have been working for weeks. You expect more.

As a result, motivation begins to wane. The intensity of your processes (the non-negotiables) reduces and your results slow down. Those early doubts you had start creeping in.

This stage will happen for everyone. I see it all the time. Any task, skill or goal that's worth achieving will have a dip, as Seth Godin explains in his book, *The Dip*.[9] You have to be self-aware enough to know you're going through it, embrace it and lean into it.

Don't shy away and take your foot off the gas in any way. That's what the dip wants you to do, and it's why so many fall at the first hurdle. You're experiencing a paradigm shift and it's time for new beginnings. Look up from the rubble, see how far you've come, reconnect with your why and start again. Trust the process and understand that the lack of instant gratification is gearing you up to enjoy the fruits of your labour afterwards.

This motivation dip will be short lived if you lean in (two to four weeks), but it could drag out if you let it get the better of you. I call it the 'grey zone' when you're in a weird range of body fat. Despite physiological fat reductions, there's no reflection of it aesthetically, and often not on the scales either.

The key here is to remain consistent in your daily processes and continue ticking your transformation checklist. What you'll find is overnight, you'll see a sudden weight drop, or you'll catch yourself in the mirror looking noticeably different, or your clothes will start fitting better. You'll know when it happens, and this is the prelude to your body kicking things up a gear in the next stage.

---

9   Godin, S (2007) *The Dip: The extraordinary benefits of knowing when to quit (and when to stick)*. Piatkus.

GATHERED MOMENTUM

It's back to the fun times again. You're seeing small wins on a weekly basis. You feel on fire, your energy is through the roof, and your body is looking better than ever. People start commenting on how well you're doing. Your confidence is building. The slog of the dip was worth it and your big vision thinking comes to the surface again.

Here's where you start pushing the pace. You want faster deadlines. This surge in gathered momentum typically lasts three to eight weeks if you stay focused on your transformation checklist. It can even go on longer. You think you're almost there, and that's when it hits you: you're back in the dip, only this time you've got different problems.

THE PRECISION DIP

No one sees this dip coming. It usually happens ten to twenty weeks into the process, but this will depend on your predicted timeframe to checkpoint.

This dip comes as a result of the fast progress you've made during stage three. With results comes complacency, and with complacency comes another roadblock to your results. By going fast and thinking you're ahead of target, you're likely skimping on the essential details. To revisit the house-build analogy for a second, the screws aren't being tightened, the pipes aren't being checked for leaks and you've picked the wrong shade of paint for the walls. It's a classic case of being close enough to your checkpoint to be able to justify not being 100% there, but far enough away to notice the impact the complacency is having, so you stall. You think your body can't get any leaner and you self-justify your behaviours. You may:

- Say yes to more social events with little to no strategy in place

- Eyeball day-to-day food instead of sticking to your meal plans

- Fall into the detrimental cycle of giving yourself permission to have or do things, telling yourself, 'I've been doing so well'

The precision dip is when you take your eye off the ball. Your level of resolve has diminished, and what starts as well-intentioned complacency can soon leave you in a rabbit hole. This is a dangerous time. Self-awareness is key here. Sticking to the processes will be your ticket to the next level.

What I like to recommend at the precision dip stage is to apply a short CTP reset to reinstall the required level of consistent intensity across all variables. One step back, two steps forward. This is especially applicable if you've grown liberal in your food choices with too much variety.

Going back to basics with your CTP accelerators for seven to fourteen days is the best way to overcome this second dip and move into the most fruitful period of the process phase, the grind. The underreporting checklist gives you eight questions to ask yourself to get you back on track.

THE RNT UNDERREPORTING CHECKLIST

✔ Have I guesstimated any of my food intake this week?

✔ Have I weighed out every single gram of my meals, including oils and seasoning?

✔ Has anything other than the meal plan passed my lips?

✔ Have I missed any of my steps, cardio or training?

✔ Am I applying the correct strategies at social events?

✔ Am I giving myself permission to do or have things that don't align with my goals?

✔ Am I being honest with what I'm reporting?

✔ Am I still checking in on time with my accountability systems (eg my coach)?

BEWARE OF THE SHINY OBJECTS

We're now living in a digital age of instant gratification and chasing dopamine hits. Whether it's an email, relationship or diet, most of us are constantly looking for what's next in our lives.

Dopamine is a brain chemical that anticipates reward. As modern society has hardwired us to chase the dopamine dragon, our ability to enjoy and cherish the reward has diminished. Instead, the reward is falling out of our hands as soon as we think we have it, so we need to catch another reward quickly to replace the looming void.

This search for the next shiny object is a problem. And the time you're most susceptible to falling into this trap is during the two dips. Earlier in this book, I discussed the four reasons you may have failed in the past to get into the shape of your life, for life. Each failure triggers a phenomenon on which the health and wellness industry thrives: programme hopping. Every time you enter a dip, you're in danger of programme hopping, especially if you haven't:

- Changed your perspective on different milestones, thinking checkpoints, not end points

- Improved your knowledge on what lies ahead of you in the next few phases of the journey

- Understood how you can achieve long-term results in the context of your lifestyle

- Spent time addressing why you're doing this

If any of the four are lacking, you're at risk. You're also not alone. We all think the grass is greener on the other side when we don't water our own. Luckily, you're reading this book, so you'll be well armed to tackle all four issues by the end.

CASE STUDY: DHINIL LEANS INTO THE DIP AND WINS

I was once guilty of the four-week rule many personal trainers live by. It's addictive. Every time I had a client who was going through the dip, I'd change the plan to spark excitement and create fake progress. It wasn't until I trained Dhinil that I started to change my ways.

An entrepreneur in his mid- to late-twenties, Dhinil had been spinning his wheels, programme hopping for years. After he'd told me more about his history and what he wanted to achieve, I decided to try a different approach.

A few months later, I remember asking myself, 'When did I last change his programme?' I checked my files and it'd been twenty weeks, but he was still getting stronger, building muscle and getting leaner. It was working like a charm, and his results spoke for themselves. Every dip he entered, we leaned into, embraced and pushed through for the rewards on the other side.

After seeing these results with Dhinil, I decided to try this approach with others. Initially they were hesitant, as I'd programmed them to grab shiny objects every time they stalled, but the results were brilliant. I began to witness the power of doubling down on one thing and focusing on execution of the process with ruthless consistency.

This is why I call phase two the process phase.

⊕ To read more about Dhinil's transformation journey, go to www.rntfitness.com/book-bonuses.

THE GRIND

What I love about the process phase is that it teaches delayed gratification. Each time you think you're close to arriving, you're faced with a new challenge to overcome, but every mini battle sets you up for your final sprint to the first checkpoint in your journey.

This is the stage of the process that gave birth to the #VaghelaGrind. The phrase was first coined a few years ago, when I was pushing a client hard to achieve a level of condition they'd always wanted. In the final few weeks, we dug deep into a place I rarely take people.

When he spoke with a friend about what my plans were with him, the friend's response was, 'You're in the Vaghela grind.' Ever since that day, the phrase has stuck at RNT to refer to the period where you press harder than you've ever done before in pursuit of your initial goal.

At the end of stage four, you'll have reconfirmed your intensity, your processes are in place again and you're firing on all cylinders. Motivation is back and at an all-time high. Your body fat is melting off and you have an ability to drive deeper into a calorie deficit to get the most out of this phase. Now is the time to pull the pin and drop the hammer.

Lower carb diets and 20,000 steps per day are common in the grind. This is when you throw the kitchen sink at your body. Don't be afraid to go to the extreme here, as it's only for a short period of time (two to four weeks). Everything you've been working on so far has been building up to this point.

You can only be in this stage if you've spent enough time in CTP and have all your processes in line. You can't expect the roof to stand strong without a stable foundation, so this is the ultimate test. It's not uncommon to see eight weeks' worth of progress happen in four, which is likely the maximum amount of time you'll be able to handle this intensity before needing a recharge break.

At this point of the process phase, you'll begin to question everything. You'll be in a place you've never been before, so remember why you're here, what's driving you, and reconnect with it – you'll need all your strength available. The aesthetic benefits are incredible, but you'll now also begin to understand the power of the physical as the vehicle for the greater good in your life.

THE FIRST TIME YOU GRIND

The first time you go through the grind is an absolute shock to the system. It's impossible to describe the feeling you have when you're in the middle of it, and the only way to understand is to experience it. A word of warning – be prepared for what's to come. It will force you into some dark places. The muck that comes up won't be easy to deal with, and it'll constantly try to drag you down and tempt you to quit.

The muck is the devil on the shoulder that will play tricks on you. It will continuously throw negative feedback loops at you: hunger, social stigmas, fatigue, mood swings, emotions – you name it. Your job is to dance with the devil, lean in and outlast it.

If it's your first time in the grind, you're likely only to see the negatives. But it's teaching you a lesson; it's actually being your friend, exposing the real battles. It's telling you what you need to work on, giving you an objective audit on your life. While you'll feel low and question whether what you're doing is healthy or normal, know the benefits are all on the other side of the grind. And it's damn well worth it.

The physical is the vehicle, and if you utilise the vehicle for all it's worth, your life will completely transform. Everyone should embrace the grind period at least once in their lives, not only for the incredible physical gains, but also for its ability to build character and resilience, and to change your life across the board. It's what separates the wheat from the chaff. It's the difference between getting into OK shape and getting into jaw-dropping shape. It's the start of a period of time in your journey that runs until the end of the next phase to shape your long-term results.

CASE STUDY: DIKSESH

A client, Diksesh, dropped 50 kg at fifty years young while running multiple businesses, overcoming numerous health problems and being an active father of two. He talked about the grind beautifully on the RNT podcast:

'I found a single-mindedness that I had never felt before in my fifty years of living. I was completely focused on the goal I had in mind and achieved a level of introspection I didn't think was possible. I must have relived every major pain point in my life. It was my "me time to callous the mind", a phrase I took from one of my favourite books *Can't Hurt Me* by David Goggins.[10] My mind was in such dark places at times that I found myself wiping the tears from my eyes while on the stair master. Everybody needs this time for introspection, to dive deep into their inner core and face all the pain they may be running away from in fear of the consequences.

'This was never about the physical. I needed to use this vehicle to live a better life doing what I love most with the people I love most. To get there, though, I needed to shed 50 kg of physical bodyweight and fifty years of mental scars carried from my childhood.

10   Goggins, D (2018) *Can't Hurt Me: Master your mind and defy the odds.* Lioncrest Publishing.

'It worked. When I reached my first checkpoint, I'd transformed from a 120 kg forty-nine-year-old man into a 71 kg fifty-year-young stud! I'd got rid of the weight of who I no longer wanted to be. It marked the peak of twelve months of brutal hard work to unlock fifty extra years of bliss. This achievement made me realise I could do anything in life.'

⊕ To hear Diksesh's powerful story, go to www.rntfitness.com/book-bonuses.

THE POWER OF THE SHOOT

The grind is one of the hardest things you'll ever do, and it will take everything you have to cross the line. You want as many levels of accountability as possible, which is why marking the transformation checkpoint with a photoshoot is powerful.

The photoshoot is never for the vanity of the pictures; it's to create a big short-term deadline, massive amounts of accountability and a memory of what you've achieved so far. It's to assess your progress, document the journey you're on, and give you a platform to build upon, reference and aim to beat in the future.

The photoshoot I had in 2019 was for this exact reason. My why was internalised and specific to the stage of my life, but the photoshoot gave me the extra accountability to embrace the process phase for what it is and never let my foot off the gas. If you know you've got a photoshoot paid for and booked in, there's no hiding. You have to face your demons right there and then and ride the rollercoaster of the process phase without falling off.

PROCESS ACCELERATORS

Before I discuss the importance, dangers and strategies of the consolidation phase, I'm going to uncover the process accelerators that will enable a smooth arrival at your first checkpoint. These accelerators are managed around your daily lifestyle commitments and challenges.

If you're busy, chances are you're going to have a lot of:

- Meals out with friends and/or family

- Networking and/or work events

- Holidays and/or business trips

Some of these events will be a breeze, whereas others will be difficult, all for different reasons:

- You may not be able to eat your required food on plan

- Your reduced willpower and hunger may get the better of you

- You may face social pressure, stigmas and scrutiny

- The process phase will expose you to these perceived negative scenarios and you need strategies to deal with them.

These are your process accelerators:

- The art of the buffer

- Social stigma armoury

- Hunger suppressors

Let's cover each accelerator in detail.

THE ART OF THE BUFFER

It's unlikely you're going to go through an entire process phase without wanting or needing to eat at a place where the ingredients and methods of cooking are out of your control. For many, this creates anxiety or panic around food options. They wonder how to continue making progress while still having a life.

No one wants to be that person pulling out a Tupperware container in a restaurant or sneaking to their car to eat their food while others wait. I say this because I've been there. I distinctly remember being in the theatre and taking out a box of tuna and vegetables. As the smell wafted into the air, I could see the disgust on everyone's faces as they turned towards me. I shrugged it off and continued eating, but it was certainly embarrassing for my family sitting next to me! There may be a time and place for such hardcore strategies, but for the most part, they're not needed.

Instead, master the art of the buffer. I call it an art because it's not black and white; it requires a process that needs fine tuning over time.

Learning how to buffer is the middle ground in a dieter's journey where you move from set meal plans and religious tracking, through guestimates and creating buffers for flexibility, to being able to autoregulate your food intake (according to your rules) in different scenarios during your week. I'll be covering the dieter's journey in more detail during the investment phase, but for now, let's focus on buffering.

WHY AND WHEN TO BUFFER

I've lost count of how many people have said to me they can't get into shape because they're too busy, they eat out too often, or – perhaps the most ridiculous – they 'only live once' and want to 'live life to the full'. The sad reality is that modern life has built social time around food and drinks, so if you're in a hard fat-loss phase, you need a strategy.

If you can avoid eating or drinking at an event and have a back-up plan in place, go for it. But this isn't always possible. Instead, building a buffer effectively saves calories for a rainy day. This can change your actions from being exclusive, where you may avoid all social events or take your own food, to inclusive, where you'll have a pre-planned buffered number of calories. In turn, this can make all the difference psychologically when you're adhering to a plan and creating a long-term lifestyle solution.

If you're wondering why we didn't cover this during phase one, it's because CTP is all about laying the foundations, removing all decisions and building non-negotiables. Aiming to work around any obstacle where possible is the best option in CTP. You'll create small wins, build confidence and generate the momentum early on which will serve you going into the process phase. You're not ready to buffer properly.

If you're in the middle of your process phase, you've got time to work a buffer in. The extent of the buffer will depend on your psychology and your timelines. If you're happy with a slow approach, you can use buffers more to keep you on track. If you're in the grind, don't even try. It's worth making the sacrifice against buffering here to stay in alignment with your goals. On the same note, if you're in a lengthy precision dip, you may need to change your buffering strategy as it could be what's holding you back.

If you're light (40–60 kg bodyweight) and/or you have a low calorie target, it'll be hard to work in regular buffers. In many cases, the buffered amount may account for your entire day's calories. This can set you backwards, so the best option is to focus on making smart choices at the event. Take charge where you can of the type of event, and if you still need to buffer, consider a two-day buffer scenario.

You also need to consider conflicting goals and actions, which comes back to realigning with your why and what type of person you want to become. As you get leaner, there's less wiggle room for buffering. If you want a typical night out or a dinner with drinks, you'll need to buffer for two to three days to make progress. Without sounding harsh, it's the reality of dieting and attempting to enjoy conflicting actions.

THE PRINCIPLES OF BUFFERING

Before implementing a buffer, understand these five rules:

- Buffering only works if you have a clear plan on how much food or drink you'll consume. You'll have a build-up of hunger, so if you're not planning ahead of time, you'll over consume.

- If you have a history of binge eating, don't buffer unless you have a clear system on how to manage your food.

- Never buffer in the evening as this is near impossible. It should be in the morning.

- If buffering in the morning creates a change in your routine meal timings, expect to feel hungrier.

- Buffers do not give you a licence to over-consume or eat calories you have not estimated for. I've seen people remove 150 to 400 calorie foods to replace them with 1,000-calorie meals, which doesn't work in the mathematics of fat loss. That's why education, and becoming aware of what and how you're eating in each phase, is so paramount here.

The first step is to do your homework on what you'll be consuming at the event. Have a plan. If the calories aren't listed online, choose something similar and make an educated guess. If you're unsure, always err on the side of caution and overestimate the calories. Never rely on your assumptions or thoughts.

Generally speaking, you're looking at 1,000 to 1,500 calories for a main meal at most restaurants. If you're adding alcohol, starters and sides on top of this, it can creep up to the 2,000 mark if you're not careful.

The second step is to remember the triggers you identified in your CTP strategy work. Even if you're armed with the best plan, buffering with trigger foods and/or in trigger environments can lead to undesired behaviour and outcomes.

The process phase is a game of mathematics and choices. Those who successfully complete a process phase while living their normal lifestyle know that buffering is a tool to be saved for when necessary. Too much of a good thing can send you backwards, so don't abuse it. Life is about choices, and you don't always need to abide by social norms to get into shape while enjoying life.

SOCIAL STIGMA ARMOURY

There comes a time during every transformation journey where you'll be ridiculed for what you're doing. It usually starts when you enter the gathered momentum stage and hits the peak during the grind. As you get into the shape of your life, the comments begin:

- You're looking too skinny

- When are you going to eat properly?

- Is this sustainable?

- You look ill

- I preferred how you looked before

It's funny because the ridicule tends to come when you least expect it. It comes when you're feeling the best you ever have, when your confidence is booming and you're expecting positive comments. If you're not ready for the opposite, it can completely throw you.

CASE STUDY: SACHIN FACES THE RIDICULE

In April 2018 I wrote an article about social stigmas that went viral over Facebook. It was sparked by a conversation with a client, Sachin:

'Akash, I need to speak to you. I don't think I can do this anymore.'

I called him up and asked what was wrong, because up till then, he'd been doing so well. He was almost forty with two young kids and sporting a body that'd make most twenty-five-year-olds jealous.

When he picked up the phone, this is what he told me:

'Everyone thinks I've gone mad. I've just come back from a wedding. My mother-in-law thinks I'm dying. My aunt asked if I'm ill. I had three of my cousins ask if everything was OK.

'My uncle said, "Enough is enough, you've shrunk and look unhealthy." What do I do? Is this normal? I've never had this before.'

'Ah, this again,' I said to myself. This wasn't the first time, and I knew it wasn't going to be the last. To this day, I have this conversation every few weeks without fail.

⊕ To read the article mentioned and learn more about Sachin's story, go to: www.rntfitness.com/book-bonuses.

Why is it that when we push the physical limits of our bodies, we get criticised in a manner that forces us to think something is wrong with us? It's time for change, and I hope this book can help.

I'd love for people to message me and say, 'Akash, I just got back from a wedding and everyone was raving about how much leaner, healthier and sharper I look. I had people asking me how I manage to look ten years younger.'

In the meantime, here's what you need to know to arm yourself against the scrutiny.

UNDERSTAND THAT IT'S DEFLECTED INSECURITIES

What's interesting is that the ones who hand out the criticism are usually deflecting their own insecurities on to you. By taking your transformation journey, you're holding up a mirror to their potential problems and issues. In fact, I've heard countless stories of the same people who dished out the criticism beginning their own journey shortly afterwards. In many cases, the critics secretly want to do what you're doing and applaud you for it, but they have no means of showing it when in social situations. This realisation is always a surprise.

EDUCATE YOUR FRIENDS, FAMILY AND PEERS

The best response you can give to the critics is to educate them on the process and tell them why it's important to you. The worst thing you can do is go into a shell, let their comments knock you down and get angry at the critics. That's what they want. Instead, appreciate their concern and explain how good you feel, your why behind your why, and how your journey is changing your life. You'll likely be surprised at the response.

REMEMBER THE BIGGER PICTURE

It's easy to think you're on the wrong path when those closest to you criticise your actions. You may even start to believe them, that you are looking too skinny. This is when it's important to remember the bigger picture. You're on a journey. You're improving yourself. You're running your own race on a path to self-mastery. Criticism is just a small road-block in the process.

HUNGER SUPPRESSORS

I regard the hunger that slowly increases over the course of the process phase as being your body's way of telling you it's burning body fat. Simplistic, I know, but it's a good mental trick to help you embrace the inevitable hunger that comes with a period of fat loss.

During the process phase you're going to be in situations where hunger is high, and you'll need strategies to help you. Whether it's to deal with social events, face day-to-day life or make the process easier, here are twelve of my best tricks:

1. Drink coffee, green and/or herbal teas

2. Eat celery sticks with black pepper

3. Take psyllium husk in between meals

4. Stay hydrated at all times

5. Drink diet fizzy drinks and/or sparkling water

6. Chew sugar-free chewing gum

7. Delay your first meal of the day

8. Plan your meal times in advance with set choices to limit decision fatigue

9. Take at least twenty minutes to eat your meals

10. Go for walks

11. Stay occupied

12. Remember your trigger, your why, your why behind your why and who you want to become in the future

Hunger is a necessary evil, but you don't need to punish yourself with it. These tricks can make arriving at your first checkpoint more enjoyable and manageable, and help you work through the challenges extra hunger may bring.

BE A LEADER

The process accelerators will transform your experience of this phase, but there's one hidden trick that obliterates all challenges and obstacles you may face in one go.

It's being a leader.

Understand that you are now in control. You have the power to make the choices that align with your highest priorities in every situation, whether it's dictating what you'll be doing with your friends and family, deciding ahead of time what your strategy is for an event, or controlling your hunger and reaction to social stigmas.

Ask yourself what would happen if:

- You organised your social plans with your friends and family for the next few months?

- You said no to the dinner and drinks networking event?

- You drank soda water with lime instead of beer when out with your friends?

- You suggested an activity-based social versus one that revolves around food and drink?

- You took charge of your choices in all situations?

Being a leader may sound scary now, but it'll grow in importance as you shift gears in the next half of the book, focusing on the 'for life' part of the equation.

BE AN ESSENTIALIST

CASE STUDY: HOW RAJ ACHIEVED MORE IN FIVE MONTHS THAN HE HAD IN FIFTEEN YEARS

In this case study, I'm going to break down how Raj worked through everything to reach his first transformation checkpoint.

Perceived struggles:

As a father of two in his mid-thirties working as an executive, Raj perceived his struggles as a lack of time, being busy and a lack of sleep. Despite training over the last few years, Raj had been unable to attain the results he craved to rid himself of the dreaded 'dad bod'.

The trigger to start:

Seeing pictures of himself with his girls and disliking how he looked.

The muck:

A lack of control of his day to day; not being clear on his priorities in life; filling his life with too much 'bloat'.

The why:

Raj wanted to stop spinning his wheels and finally achieve the body he'd been working hard to attain for fifteen years.

The why behind the why:

To be a high performer at work, be present with his family and inspire his girls to live a healthy and productive lifestyle.

Long-term vision:

To be someone who values their health and fitness, identifies with a lean lifestyle, and is able to inspire others around him to do the same.

First checkpoint timeframe:

Raj's first checkpoint was to get into the shape of his life in a timeframe of between sixteen and twenty weeks.

Accountability systems:

Raj ensured he had all three levels of accountability covered:

- **Self** – he continued to remind himself why he was doing this and the long-term vision of who he was becoming.

- **Peer** – after experiencing social stigmas, Raj explained his journey to those around him and gained the support he needed from his family and friends.

- **Coach** – Raj is the perfect client who checks in on time every week with everything we need to work our magic.

- **Bonus** – in stage four of the process phase, the precision dip, Raj added another layer of accountability by booking in a photoshoot to mark his transformation checkpoint.

3Ss:

Raj's 3Ss were designed around tackling his perceived struggles:

- **Structure** – the key for Raj was building a sustainable structure that worked around his job and his girls' schedules. This meant waking up earlier to get steps in and planning his weeks in advance to install his non-negotiables in his diary without fail.

- **System** – given his daily responsibilities, Raj needed a system that was decision free, especially around his diet. He also needed to tackle two perceived problems of time to complete steps and a lack of sleep. This meant walking calls and meetings, altered commute routes and having a treadmill at home so he could walk while keeping an eye on the children. These were big wins that built confidence in creating a real lifestyle solution.

- **Strategy** – with endless networking and client entertainment events, along with regular holidays with family and friends, Raj became a master of buffering and managing his hunger in different environments.

Initial transformation checklist:

- **Training** – four days a week on a structured progressive overload-focused programme

- **Nutrition** – 1,700 calories with around 160 g protein, 60 g fat and 120 g carbohydrate

- **Steps** – 10,000 steps per day

- **Water** – 3 litres per day

- **Sleep** – seven unbroken hours was the aim, although the key was improving the quality of the sleep he got due to the unpredictable sleep habits of his children

Honeymoon period:

With the 3Ss locked in and the foundation laid, Raj was en route to finally cracking the code for his body.

Motivation dip:

In the first six weeks of his journey, Raj saw minimal movement on the scales despite his whole physique changing dramatically. He was losing body fat, but the metrics weren't picking it up. Because Raj was being consistent with his transformation checklist for the first time in fifteen years, he was building muscle, which skewed the scale metrics further. Given his preconceived associations linking the scales to success, he was thrown, adding frustration to the process.

Gathered momentum:

After staying true to his 3Ss and ticking off the transformation checklist every day, Raj pulled out of the grey zone and racked up a lot of small wins.

Precision dip:

Despite knowing the benefits of limiting decision fatigue, Raj began to flirt with excessive variety using different food tracking apps. The problem was that this was eating away at his willpower, making adhering to the social, work and holiday strategies he had in place more difficult. He applied a CTP reset, booked a photoshoot and entered the grind.

The grind:

In the final four weeks before his photoshoot, Raj pushed the intensity of his transformation checklist with over 15,000 steps a day and the addition of zero carb days. Reflecting on this period, Raj said:

'I had, up until now, achieved small wins and built up habits, which had given me the momentum and the confidence to enter the grind. I felt that if I could nail this period, I could tackle anything else further down the line.

'I began to wake up at 4–5am on days when the kids slept through and opted to go on the treadmill rather than outdoors to do my cardio. This meant I could keep the baby monitor beside me in case my younger daughter woke up. When I needed to take the train to work, I would walk to and from the local station rather than taking the car, and I'd get off the train a stop earlier than I needed. I did a lot of walking calls and opted to go for walks after dinner to binge on the RNT catalogue of podcasts. All these small changes contributed to the calorie deficit I was building up. My training sessions were still non-negotiable, I was meal prepping to limit decisions, and I had a super-supportive wife who put up with everything the grind brings with it.'

Raj's grind insights:

When I asked Raj what his greatest insight was during the grind, he replied, 'I learnt the power of essentialism.'

In love with his answer, I asked him to elaborate.

'When you're tired, low on energy and running on fumes, you have no choice but to highlight the essential and cut out all the bloat. I started asking myself:

- What should I spend my time doing?

- What do I want to do with my limited energy?

- Who should I spend my limited time and energy on and with?

'When the gas tank is low, you can't waste your precious resources on anything.'

Transformation checkpoint:

Pushing through the grind led to the transformation checkpoint that Raj had been working towards for fifteen years. He was in the shape of his life with unshakeable confidence. He was also a step closer to his big why of leading a healthy lifestyle to inspire his girls.

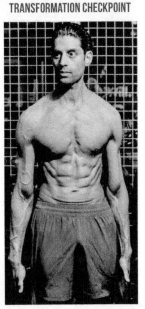

BEFORE   TRANSFORMATION CHECKPOINT

⊕ To read more about Raj's journey to his first checkpoint and beyond, go to www.rntfitness.com/book-bonuses.

In becoming an essentialist, you debate some of life's most difficult questions. You ask the questions you may have been putting off, struggling with, or afraid to know the real answer to:

- What do I want out of my life, my relationships and my career?

- How do I want to live my day to day?

- Am I willing to make the sacrifices in specific areas of life to push in other areas?

- What truly drives me?

- What do I enjoy doing, and what do I hate?

It's the equivalent of spring cleaning all areas of your life. A client, Puja, summed it up perfectly:

> 'There's no hiding in this process. Everything you need to work on comes up, as if you're stirring a well. All the dirt at the bottom of the well comes up to the top, and you realise how much you need to clean the water before you drink it.'

In stirring up the well on limited resources, you understand the escape or coping mechanisms you've held on to as a crutch to deal with your muck. It could be drink, drugs, partying, food, sex, work, travel and so on. Everyone has them.

CASE STUDY: PUJA'S CRUTCH

For Puja, her crutch resided in food. A woman in her mid-thirties coming out of a difficult marriage, she viewed food as her only source of comfort. It was her way to deal with all the stress and anxiety of the split.

Over the years, she found herself gaining 25 kg of excess bodyweight. Identifying the muck for Puja was easy; keeping her self-aware enough to know when she was slipping into old habits and abandoning her 3Ss was the difficult task.

In reality, she'd outgrown the need for food as a source of comfort. Going through the grind for Puja meant shedding the skin of her old self and rebuilding herself from the start again.

The grind teaches you the reality of true hunger signals. It's common to eat because of social norms, habit and boredom. You hear stories all the time of people eating mindlessly at work, at home, in front of the TV or in social situations. The grind exposes this and makes you question your feelings of boredom in parts of your life.

Because of that looming checkpoint, you can't eat mindlessly anymore. There's too much at stake, which can be life changing in itself. It never surprises me when people make bold decisions with their careers and relationships during or shortly after a grind phase.

CASE STUDY: TIM

Tim, a writer and executive in Toronto, experienced this exact phenomenon after losing nearly 25 kg on his way to his first checkpoint:

'I remember during the grind it dawned on me that I had been using socialising as a gateway to 4,000-calorie evenings of drinks and food. This journey exposed my bad habits and practices that I'd normalised. When your transformation checklist becomes demanding, your whole life goes under audit, from your relationships to your career, your social time – everything. It's incredible the small changes you can make in your life as a result that can lead to massive benefits forever.'

To explore Puja and Tim's life-changing stories in full, go to www.rntfitness.com/book-bonuses.

Exercise: Have you had your aha moment?

As we approach the halfway mark of the book, I want you to ask yourself if you've had an aha moment. Has the lightbulb with the hidden lifestyle solution gone off in your head yet?

Every one of you will have had one specific struggle that caused you to pick this book up and find a solution. It's why you've always failed to achieve your long-term goals.

If your head is flashing and screaming aha, write it down. If not, keep an eye out as we step into the uncharted territory of consolidation. It may be waiting for you there.

TRANSFORMATION CHECKPOINT

You've made it. You've reached your first goal. Your house is built.

You look great, you feel great, you've conquered many of the demons, insecurities and struggles of your past. You're in the shape of your life. What's next?

The first step is to reconnect with your past failures and remember why this time will be different. Think checkpoint, not the end. Think journey, not a one-off plan. Think about the big-picture goal you have here: the new identity you want to create and the muck from your past you want to continue to shed. Your past failures are there to remind you that this is when the hard work begins.

At this stage, ask yourself:

- How can you look and feel even better?

- How do you hold on to the sense of accomplishment instead of repeating old failures?

- How do you stay in the shape of your life, for life?

The answer lies in the critical period of the next phase, consolidation. However many weeks you've spent pushing to this checkpoint, you need to add four to twelve more so you can safely consolidate and set yourself up for a long-term lifestyle solution.

SUMMARY

Goal:

- Focus on daily processes to achieve your transformation checkpoint

Process essentials:

- Honeymoon period

- Motivation dip

- Gathered momentum

- Precision dip

- The grind

Process accelerators:

- The art of the buffer

- Social stigma armoury

- Hunger suppressors

Now it's time for a new beginning. It's time to think beyond this first checkpoint and uncover the strategies required to build on your progress. It's time to start the hard work.

That may sound crazy after the grind you've just finished, but it's the reality. Working towards the first checkpoint is easy in comparison. A well-executed consolidation phase serves as the lynchpin, connecting your initial goals with gains over a long period of time. Everything you've done so far has primed you for what's to come.

Now you've reached your transformation checkpoint, let's look at how you can maintain what you've worked so hard to build in the next phase, consolidation.

4
PHASE THREE: CONSOLIDATION

The aim of the consolidation phase is to maintain everything you've achieved so far. It's the critical period that many fail in. A well-executed consolidation phase can set you up for long-term success in building the lifestyle solutions required to stay in shape.

This is where the hard work begins.

CASE STUDY: MY FAILURE

In 2014 I made a crucial mistake. I'd just competed in and won my first bodybuilding show after seventeen weeks of dieting where I lost 13 kg and achieved my best-ever condition.

I remember it vividly – Sunday 27 July. It was the only date I'd had in mind for seventeen weeks straight. As the date came closer, the hunger, the cravings, the social stigmas all appeared, but I kept saying to myself, 'Four weeks to go', 'Fifteen days left' and, worst of all, 'I can't wait to eat pizza, chips and burgers again.' With a singular focus on 27 July, I stocked up on all my favourite foods, watched food programmes whenever I had free time, and thought about all the things I could do from 28 July.

I was gearing up for absolute disaster. As soon as I won my competition, I ate all the foods I'd stocked up on, visited three restaurants in the first twenty-four hours and was packing my suitcase for an all-inclusive holiday in Greece. Seven days later, I was 7 kg heavier and a mess. If you'd seen me on 3 August, you'd never have known I'd picked up a bodybuilding trophy just one week before.

Fast forward another six weeks and I was a total of 14 kg up from my leanest. I was worse than back to square one. It was embarrassing.

This story is a big part of why I'm writing this book: I don't want anyone else to experience the same. What followed was a year of yo-yoing, spinning my wheels and lacking any perspective or knowledge on what I should do. Up till 27 July, I'd thought getting into bodybuilding condition was difficult, but the twelve months of struggle that came after were brutal. I didn't expect the struggle. I had neither direction nor preparation.

While it was an unpleasant experience, this period of my life taught me valuable lessons. I don't want to repeat it myself, nor see any of my clients experience it. When I finally climbed out of this rut at the tail end of 2015, I became obsessed with the consolidation phase.

The lynchpin of the transformation journey, the consolidation phase is the difference between regression and progression. It's the critical period that you need to master if you want to get into the shape of your life, for life. It will prime you for the investment and reward phases to come. Without it, you'll soon be back at the beginning, like I was.

Since starting RNT, I've spoken more about the consolidation phase on articles, podcasts and videos than anything. And my obsession with this phase means I've never repeated the experience of 2014. When I next competed in July 2017, I was a different person as I reversed out of the extreme low body fat with ease. At my photoshoot in 2019, it was even better. It was effortless.

Perhaps more rewarding is how my clients have experienced this journey. Before understanding the importance of consol- idation, my clients would rebound horrifically. All my industry friends were having the same problem with their clients, which was why creating a consolidation phase for everyone to go through was vital. With all the coaching, content and conversations around consolidation, my team and I at RNT are able to facilitate our clients to achieve the shape of their lives – and learn how to keep it.

I'm going to tell you how to do the same now. To begin with, I'm going to discuss the critical first steps to take, before outlining the consolidation accelerators that will make navi- gating through this phase as seamless as possible.

AVOIDING THE REBOUND

If I reflect back on 2014, my failures stemmed from the four reasons I outlined at the start of this book:

- I had a lack of correct perspective, believing 27 July was the end.

- I had a lack of knowledge of what to do after 27 July and no idea of what I could achieve.

- I didn't believe I could maintain my results and build upon what I'd achieved while still having a life.

- I had a lack of clear underpinnings for getting into the shape of my life and why it was important to me.

I had no plan, no preparation and no purpose. Mentally, I was set up for failure.

The body likes homeostasis, so when we take it away from its natural set point, it will fight with us to go back to normal. If we dive deeper into the science here, it's important to understand that when we reduce body fat, we don't reduce the number of fat cells. They just shrink in size.

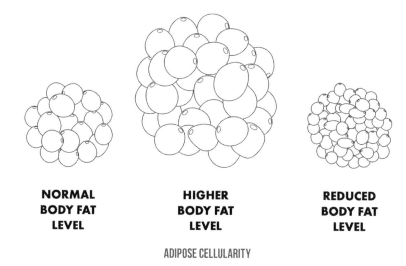

| NORMAL BODY FAT LEVEL | HIGHER BODY FAT LEVEL | REDUCED BODY FAT LEVEL |

ADIPOSE CELLULARITY

The problem is that shrunken fat cells will always be ready and waiting to fill up again if we quickly enter a calorie excess. This is why it's so easy to yo-yo after a diet. Our body is primed to return to previous body fat levels where its homeostatic place is, or worse yet, higher fat levels.

That's not the only bad news, though. Depending on how quickly you gain body fat, not only will you fill your original fat cells back up, but your body will create even more. This is why people struggle dieting for the second time after having rebounded – they now have 10–20% more fat cells. They may be smaller fat cells, but there are more of them and they're more spread out.

It gets worse. Smaller fat cells have less leptin (a hormone that tells you when you're full) and they're more sensitive to insulin (a storage hormone). This means even if you're eating more, you're constantly hungry *and* more prone to storing body fat. That's why in the six weeks following 27 July 2014,

I ended up in a worse position than I'd started in and found it hard to get back into shape.

There are also psychological effects of the rebound. You'll see poor relationships with food develop, low confidence and possibly even mild forms of depression. I experienced all these in 2014.

The good news is that a well-executed consolidation phase can help you avoid these problems. In fact, mastering this critical period will highlight to you the power of the physical to act as the vehicle to the greater good in your life. By controlling your emotions and psychology and your body's physiology, even when they're all fighting against you, you'll develop a level of self-confidence that exceeds the euphoria of your first transformation checkpoint. You'll be one step closer to self-mastery.

REMOVING THE ANTICLIMAX

The end of the process phase can feel like an anticlimax when you wake up the next day. You've poured everything into the grind, taken yourself to the extreme, and you may now be feeling a bit lost. Before, the checkpoint was so close and clear. You knew what the initial goal was, and every week you had tangible results to reward your efforts. Now, what's to keep you ticking the boxes of your transformation checklist? Why shouldn't you eat the boxful of doughnuts? The mind games are going to be tough and, the first time, unlike anything you've experienced.

That's why the first step to take after you reach your transformation checkpoint is to reconnect with your long-term vision, your plan and your why. In 2014, I had none of these foundations and my new house came crashing down. By taking this first step, you'll remove the anticlimax and think of the future. You'll remember why this was only a checkpoint, a necessary step to achieve what you truly want. Remember why you picked this book up. Everything you've learnt thus far is to prime you for the next half of the equation: getting in shape *for life*.

BATTLING THE CONSOLIDATION MIND GAMES

Your body will be fighting you. It will be calling for food, hunger will be high and you will have triggers everywhere. That's why you must maintain the same structure, strategy and system that helped you build your new house in the first place. You need to solidify the cement; the bricks you've laid down aren't set yet. It's a dangerous time and you're not quite ready to move into the house yet.

I know how tempting it is to want to add in excessive variety, change and/or luxury at this point. Don't. Keep it basic. Maintain your 3Ss. Stick with your CTP accelerators. And know that if you can spend six to eight weeks letting the cement dry, you can move into your new house safely and start planning for life.

That's exciting. That's when you can add more variety, use more flexible social strategies and consume more palatable foods without being triggered. Until then, keep in mind that your psychology and physiology are working against you. They will tell you to eat. They will justify your self-sabotage. The control that you've worked hard to build in the process phase will completely go if you're not careful. Solidify the cement.

This doesn't only happen to a select few. I've been there multiple times. I've seen hundreds of others fall prey to this too. It is the trait of someone who's been through a period of fat loss.

CONSOLIDATION CTP RESET

The best way to battle the mind games of consolidation is to stick by your 3Ss, reconnect with your long-term vision and think of your why. This will empower you with the freedom to maintain control in this critical period. A fourteen- to twenty-one-day CTP, albeit with a higher amount of quality calories, is the recipe for success here.

This is your consolidation CTP reset. Limit your decisions, tighten your non-negotiables and practise your precursors daily. By doing so, you'll avoid the temptation for 'one more', the tendency to 'try a little of this' or the self-justification of 'I've worked hard so deserve that'. There's a time and place for all of this, but it shouldn't be a regular feature of the consolidation phase.

After fourteen to twenty-one days of the consolidation CTP reset, you'll have a better control of your feedback signals from your psychology and physiology. You can then add more variety, create extra freedom and test the waters with new foods and situations. You still want to tread carefully, though, and wait for the six- to eight-week period to finish before making any significant shift in your approach.

IS YOUR TRANSFORMATION CHECKLIST STILL APPLICABLE?

The non-negotiable processes you created in the CTP phase and focused on in the process phase will always be fundamental to what you do. Your intensity, direction and ability to autoregulate each non-negotiable will depend on the phase you're in.

By the end of the process phase, you will have pushed your transformation checklist to a hard level with lower calories, harder training and higher step targets. It's tempting to drop the ball on everything after the transformation checkpoint, and that's what the consolidation CTP reset is there for. By keeping your 3Ss in place, you can now dial the intensity down over the course of six to eight weeks. Depending on how your body reacts in this time, slowly increase calories, reduce activity and train less often to the point of failure. Your body will have been through a lot, so now isn't the time to go all guns blazing. At the same time, it's not the time to stop doing everything. That'd be a fast way to undo all your hard work.

CONSOLIDATION ACCELERATORS

Even with the best intentions of removing the anticlimax, applying a consolidation CTP reset, fighting the mind games and systematically reducing the intensity of your transformation checklist, you will need consolidation accelerators to maximise your chance of success:

- Developing meal hygiene

- Shifting from an aesthetic to performance mindset

- Maintaining your accountability systems

Let's take a closer look at each one.

DEVELOPING MEAL HYGIENE

As we get further into the second half of the book, we'll be questioning many of the old habits and automatic daily actions you may take for granted. They may have even been contributors to your previous failures. The first is your level of meal hygiene.

Meal hygiene refers to your mindset and behaviours towards food, as well as your ability to create a healthy relationship around your eating practices. Ask yourself these questions:

- Are you the first one to finish at the dinner table?

- Do you finish meals so stuffed you can't move?

- Are you failing to put your knife and fork down between bites?

- Do you ever finish a meal and wonder whether it tasted good?

- When in social settings, are you so focused on your plate that you don't engage with your companions?

- Do you feel bloated and gassy after you eat?

- Are you in a rush when you eat?

If you're answering yes to most of the above, you have poor meal hygiene. The consequences are:

- Lack of satiety from your meals

- Poor relationship with food

- Inability to control food portions

- Lack of self-awareness around foods you actually like and dislike

- Poor social engagement when eating with peers

- Digestion problems

- Higher likelihood to overeat

Meal hygiene is something you've likely not paid attention to in the past. It's not spoken about, and it's often so engrained into our daily habits, we don't even think about it. It's generally something we develop as a child.

Do you remember your parents telling you to 'Make sure you clear your plate' or 'Hurry up and finish your food'? I know mine did. They meant well, but the subconscious food behaviours, associations and habits we've developed as a result can be damaging if we don't tune into them.

In an increasingly fast and digital world, meal hygiene is a topic that needs special attention to help us maintain self-awareness, mindfulness and a healthy relationship with food. Poor meal hygiene can highlight the psychological and physiological problems during the consolidation phase and make them worse. It will come to light in an inability to control ourselves around food. All the engrained habits we've spent decades automating will lead us astray here as they feed the body's desire for food, fast.

The good news is that I'm going to share the RNT meal hygiene checklist.

RNT MEAL HYGIENE CHECKLIST

- ✔ Eat all meals without any devices in front of you
- ✔ Take ten deep breaths before consuming any meals
- ✔ Aim for twenty+ chews per mouthful
- ✔ Put your knife and fork down between mouthfuls
- ✔ Move away from your work station when eating
- ✔ Try expressing gratitude before meals
- ✔ Eat at a designated eating area for all meals
- ✔ Where possible, don't eat on the move
- ✔ Stay present when eating; feel the different textures and flavours
- ✔ Set aside at least fifteen to twenty minutes per meal to ensure you aren't rushing

Think about how many items on the RNT meal hygiene checklist you can tick off and where you're lacking. For your next meal, implement one missing tip and notice how you feel. I'd expect you to have a more satisfying and enjoyable meal, with a heightened taste experience. If you've got company, expect more engaging conversation and connection. It's a win-win.

Scoring well on the RNT meal hygiene checklist also correlates with maintaining lean behaviours and healthy condition year-round.

THE FOOD WILL ALWAYS BE THERE

A liberating shift in thinking at this stage is to take the pressure away from fear of missing out. If you've come out of the grind, it's easy to slip into the mindset of 'I need to make up for lost time'. Don't.

A better approach is to remind yourself that the food will always be there. It's not going anywhere. If you find yourself slipping, check yourself and remember that there will always be another opportunity to eat. Stay present and calm, adopt strong meal hygiene and be grateful for what you have in front of you.

CASE STUDY: KUNAAL'S GELATO TEMPTATION

The perfect example here is Nairobi-based entrepreneur, Kunaal. After losing over 20 kg bodyweight and 25 cm off his waist, he wanted to 'make up for lost time' by eating his wife's delicious homemade gelato.

With a small factory at home for his wife's business, Kunaal had to be careful. Once he realised the danger of his thinking after a few slip-ups, Kunaal changed his strategy. He started incorporating one scoop of gelato every evening into his calories, eating it with good meal hygiene. Any urges to overeat disappeared as he learnt moderation. While there was always more he could eat, he discovered how to enjoy the texture, taste and experience of the food versus mindlessly eating.

⊕ To read Kunaal's journey, go to www.rntfitness. com/book-bonuses.

A GRADUAL SHIFT AWAY FROM BUFFERING

One of the key strategies that I talked about in the process phase was learning the art of buffering to navigate around occasions where you can't always control your food intake. Once you're out of the initial fourteen to twenty-one days of the consolidation CTP reset, buffering is something I want you to think about moving away from. That's not to say you disregard it, but reconsider the potentially aggressive buffers you may have used in the process phase.

The consolidation phase is when you learn:

- How to exercise impromptu portion control

- Nutritional values, labels and contents, increasing your education

- What foods you like and dislike

This starts with developing meal hygiene. As you're now more mindful around your food, you'll be able to tune in to the psychological (cravings and a 'need to eat' mentality) and physiological (hunger and satiety) receptors that are recovering back to normal after the fourteen- to twenty-one-day consolidation CTP reset, and even more noticeably after the six- to eight-week mark. The wide variety in timeframes here covers the differences in how each individual's feedback mechanisms recover.

Up until your transformation checkpoint, you may have let the autopilot of your 3Ss carry you to the top. I want you to keep this autopilot switched on but dim it down to 80% of the time. In the 20% zone, experiment with new foods while using meal hygiene practices to understand:

- Which foods you eat quickly and which foods you like to eat slowly and enjoy.

- How long it takes for you to feel full if you follow good meal hygiene.

- What associations you notice with different foods. Are there any foods that trigger specific emotions?

- Which foods you enjoy and which foods you don't actually like. This question surprises many people.

Focus on building self-awareness around your food and continue tracking most of it so you can build the knowledge from the ground up on what food looks like as a raw weight. Using the 20% zone, learn the difference between 250 g potatoes and 50 g rice, not only in appearance, but also in satiety, hunger and enjoyment, despite both containing a similar amount of carbohydrates.

This variety can extend to different cooking methods, which in turn will help you see how food looks in restaurants versus at home. Ask yourself:

- What cooking methods are used?

- What has the food been cooked in?

- Are the portion sizes much bigger or smaller than when you cook at home? If they're different, how do the calories stack up when you consider the little things they've added, eg sauces, oil for cooking, seasoning, etc?

Take mental notes of any disparities here against your baseline education of single-ingredient cooking weighed out to the gram.

This practice is something buffering will have taught you to an extent, but you now want to be in a position where buffering isn't necessary. You can go out, enjoy a meal and know you won't overeat or overspill your daily calories. You can live life and still be in shape. It sounds simple, but this is where you may have slipped up in the past, which is why the consolidation phase is the lynchpin. Value this time as the connecting phase to your long-term success.

SHIFTING FROM AN AESTHETIC TO PERFORMANCE MINDSET

You have your long-term vision of who you want to be. You know how the physical will act as a vehicle to facilitate this. At the same time, humans thrive off short-term goals to help steer the ship in the right direction. Until your transformation checkpoint, your short-term goals will have been aesthetically driven as your main progress indicators will have been bodyweight loss per week, measurements and, ultimately, your appearance.

The consolidation phase brings with it new goals. So far, we've discussed a number of new practices, approaches and mindsets to help you use this critical period as a primer for your future phases. The problem you may find is that it's all intangible and difficult to track objectively. That's where the power of performance indicator targets comes into play.

You now shift your mindset from being physique oriented to performance based, focusing on strength over aesthetics.

As we know, strength is the best indicator of muscle retention and gain, and overall physique development. But from now on, it becomes your driving tangible indicator. In the consolidation phase, you want to create this shift in mindset.

MAINTAINING YOUR ACCOUNTABILITY SYSTEMS

Reflecting on 2014, I realised another critical mistake I'd made that came from ignorance. I removed all my accountability systems – I stopped taking regular pictures, discontinued working with my coach and took the bodyweight scales away from my daily check-ins. I rode the success train of having won a bodybuilding show to tell everyone around me it was 'all back to normal living now'. It was a heavy price that I paid for my lack of knowledge.

Of all the above, removing the scales and lack of pictures hurt me the most. After weighing in after my all-inclusive holiday at 7 kg more than I'd been a week prior, I didn't weigh myself or take pictures for another six weeks. I kidded myself into thinking I was gaining muscle, looking well and that scale weight didn't matter. Had I been armed with the right knowledge, I'd have known about the objectivity scale weight and pictures can provide in a time when I was at my most subjective with myself.

Your ability to self-justify is so high when you reach your transformation checkpoint that listening to your internal voice is futile, especially if you've never successfully been through a consolidation phase. Weighing yourself and taking pictures regularly will keep you honest and accountable.

If I review my more recent consolidation phases and those of people who effortlessly walk through this phase – often on their first time – I realise we realign our long-term vision while maintaining all the accountability systems that took us to the first transformation checkpoint. This period can create a genuine fear of accountability, as such systems will force us to exert control in our behaviour and practices, which can be uncomfortable for some. It's easy to run and hide.

I felt like that in 2014. I stopped using my coach because I was too scared to face the reality. Bad mistake. All it led to was failure and disappointment. I missed out on another layer of objective accountability, where I could have discussed, monitored and tweaked my 3Ss in accordance with my psychology and body's response. I'd have known what rate of fat gain was acceptable, whether my food behaviours were normal, or if I was crossing the line of eating bad food for the sake of it. I was lost and didn't know any of the answers but was too afraid to confront the reality. My mistakes have taught me the best strategy here is to embrace the difficulty and lean into it.

DON'T PUNISH YOURSELF

The consolidation phase will be a rocky period full of mind games, emotions and mental battles as you fight to gain control of your body's psychological and physiological feed-back mechanisms. Even if you're armed with all the best strategies to master the consolidation phase, you will have a few moments of weakness. That's OK. Don't punish yourself by dieting. All this will do is teach your habit systems to diet after every moment of weakness, while compounding the yo-yo mentality you're trying to remove. Instead, identify the triggers that cause you to derail.

Remember the goal of this phase is to transition from focusing hard on the processes required to get into the shape of your life to priming you to learn the strategies that will help you stay there. Be kind to yourself. If you mess up, enjoy it, own it and move on as normal at the next opportunity. There's always a chance to get better, and each time you go off track, use it as a learning to know what you shouldn't do next time. Ask yourself why it happened. Dig deeper. Think of the bigger picture. Become self-aware in every situation you put yourself in and build an education bank you can utilise in the future.

The consolidation phase is where you'll begin to understand the power of controlling your physical body in its most fragile state. This builds confidence. Harness it. Know that if you can get through this, the sky is the limit with what you can achieve.

IT GETS EASIER EVERY TIME

Just like the first grind is a shock to the system, your first consolidation phase will be similar. As much as I can give you the strategies to solidify the cement of your new house, it will be difficult. It might be one of the hardest things you'll do. You will learn about yourself in a way you've not been exposed to before.

The one aspect that can be most hard to wrap your head around is knowing that your body will fight everything you do. At the same time, you have to tune into your body with self-awareness to override thwarted hunger and satiety signals. This takes real skill. The first time will always be tough, but it does get easier every time.

In 2014, I was a rookie with no plan. In 2017, I was ten times better because I had a plan. In 2019, I became a consolidation master and was in complete control of everything.

When you start controlling the narrative of your body, you'll be able to hide all the noise that its signals are emitting and focus on what it truly needs. The key to success here is knowing what's coming, creating a plan and realigning with your long-term purpose. Remember the four reasons for failure and use everything this book has taught you so far to win this phase.

CASE STUDY: FIRST-TIME CHAMPIONS

This chapter has brought many of my own struggles with consolidation to the surface. It's been the hardest phase for me to conquer; I took five years to get to grips with it. But my pain has been RNT clients' gain, and it's rare now to witness a failed consolidation. Every week my team and I are seeing first timers to the RNT journey dominate this critical period and set themselves up for a productive investment phase.

Adam, a serial entrepreneur who'd always struggled to stay in shape after dieting, recalls his first consolidation:

'As an ex rugby player, I was super fit and strong, regularly "winning" the CrossFit workouts in my local gym. I was training six days a week and feeling great. But I didn't look in shape like the other guys.

'In truth, I'd constantly yo-yoed over the past ten years between looking good and stocky. There was a consistent 5–20 kg swing in bodyweight on a regular basis. I wanted to change this. I wanted to first get into the shape of my life, and then learn how to stay there.

'Running multiple successful businesses means I have to be on my triple A game at all times. I know how crucial it is for my mind and body to be functioning well to be a high performer. The biggest game changers for me were:

- Building my education database of food, through learning what foods contained what, how they made me feel, and which were my triggers.

- Learning and practising meal hygiene. This was the aha moment I'd been searching for all these years. I was the classic guy who'd finish two rounds at the buffet before most had even started their first plate. Slowing down gave me a new sense of satisfaction that enabled me to maintain control during the vulnerable time of consolidation.'

Tej, an investment professional based in London who regularly works sixteen+ hours a day, mastered her first consolidation phase, building herself a plat-form to create a lifestyle solution to effortlessly stay in shape year-round. With a daunting schedule filled with networking events, work drinks, socials and high-stress deadlines, she had enough excuses to throw anyone off the rails after reaching her trans-formation checkpoint. Eighteen months on, I asked her what her secret was to staying exactly the same bodyweight.

'I can put it down to three keys:

- I know who I want to be. I want to be someone who is healthy and lean, and takes care of themselves all the time. I have every excuse to go off track, but the benefits of staying in the shape of my life, for life to my career, confidence and mental health are immeasurable.

- I used to over-indulge at socials, work drinks or networking events. Now I consciously choose the best options and shift my focus from the food to being present.

- I aim to avoid using food or drink as a social vehicle as much as I can. There are so many more interesting ways to collaborate with family, friends and colleagues.'

Dhaval, a leading dermatologist and medical professional from New York City, lost over 20 kg and has kept it off. Twelve months later, he said:

'I travel, on average, twice a week to speak at conferences or attend meetings. I'm often at hotels that don't serve the limited food options I can eat because I'm vegetarian. It's crucial I make good choices where I can.

'The physical is the vehicle for me to lead from the front with my patients, perform at my optimum and have the energy to work eighteen hours a day running my different businesses and projects. I keep this in mind at all times, hold myself accountable at all three levels, focus on performance and understand that this is a long-term play.'

⊕ To hear more of Adam, Tej and Dhaval's stories, go to www.rntfitness.com/book-bonuses.

MASTERING THE TIP OF THE MOUNTAIN

The period of approximately twelve weeks from the start of the grind (phase two, stage five) to the end of consolidation becomes the definitive time for how the rest of your journey plays out. Imagine yourself climbing to the summit of Mount Kilimanjaro. All throughout the process phase, you'll have encountered sharp hills and small downturns; big rocks and small rocks; edgy rocks and sharp rocks; rocks of all shapes and sizes. You'll have tripped a few times, taken a few beatings and doubted whether you'll ever be able to get to the top.

As you approach the summit, despite being hungry, thirsty and tired, you grind. You climb faster than ever with energy you never thought you had. You're able to dig deeper than you imagined. You should be beat, but the opportunity to plant your flag at the top of the mountain trumps everything. Your focus is relentless; your commitment to the cause is unwavering; you've come so far on this journey that turning back is no longer an option. The summit is within reach.

When you reach the top, you plant your flag, mark your checkpoint and absorb the incredible panoramic views. The blood, sweat and tears you have put in have all been worth it. The doubters are silenced, the path you took is vindicated and you achieve something only a few manage.

At this point you have three options. The first is to stay at the top and milk it for what it's worth, before realising there's limited oxygen. This is the path of the perpetual dieter – someone who forms an unhealthy relationship with food intake, becomes obsessed with dieting and believes that it's impossible to stay in shape while living life.

The second is to find the fastest route home, accepting all risk and falling down every 100 metres. The injuries accumulate, and by the time you're back at the bottom, you wish you'd never even started the climb. You're in worse shape than when you started, both physically and mentally, just like my own 2014 story.

This option is the most common because of:

- A lack of knowledge on what to do next and how exactly to climb down from the summit. The map or guides you used to get to the top have now disappeared, and the paths and terrains you came up on don't exist anymore. It's a different road back with plenty of thorns, ditches and gaps to make it a new challenge altogether. Most fail because they forget this, or aren't aware in the first place.

- Overconfidence from the results so far. The same people who criticised you on the way up are now praising you, and with this comes a belief that you're invincible. As a result, you lose control of your food (ie binge) and think nothing bad will come of it.

In most cases, it's a combination of both.

The third option is to take the safe passage home, the road less taken. It's not the fastest, the smoothest or the easiest, but it's the path that'll bring you back in one piece and allow you to maintain the same feeling and shape as you had at the top. You may have a few scuffs, but no long-term injuries or surgery required.

This is the well-executed consolidation phase. It's what puts you in a prime position to invest in the next phase and enable a real lifelong transformation. You won't need to diet again; you can invest long term and win the second half of your equation, preparing for the next adventure.

Those who succeed here will have thought about consolidation all throughout the grind and planned it out beforehand. These people know that reaching the top of the mountain is easy. They know better than to let go of the map and the guide at the summit, which is when they need them the most.

When you take the safe passage home, the aesthetic benefit is that you'll be in much better condition at the same altitude. When you reverse in a sensible, strategic manner, you will look so much better than you did at the same weight when you started the grind. All of this together breeds an unmatched level of confidence. You'll have mastered your mind and body, and now you'll have the confidence to master anything.

CASE STUDY: EVERYTHING COMES TOGETHER FOR RAJ

In the last chapter, we explored Raj's journey to his transformation checkpoint. What happened next was where everything came together for him. In the six to eight weeks after the grind, he conquered consolidation despite facing the challenge of two weeks on an all-inclusive family trip to Disneyland and Antigua.

'I had prepared for consolidation well in advance of the transformation checkpoint. My coach hammered it down my throat, I knew what was coming and what I wanted in the long term, so failure wasn't an option. I took the safe passage home and used all the consolidation accelerators given to me, despite many changes in environment.

'Having dealt with the social stigmas and the crazy hunger signals near the peak of the summit to beat all the demons that come with the initial return down, I felt unstoppable. The productive investment phase I'm in now would never have been possible if I hadn't smashed through the grind, hit my check-point and conquered consolidation. This trio has been critical for me. I came out of my consolidation phase at roughly the same bodyweight as I was when entering the grind, but aesthetically, I looked so much better for it. What my coach refers to as the tip of the mountain could not be a more critical period for anyone on their journey.'

Mastering the tip of the mountain is the ultimate form of self-control. Sanjeeta, who I introduced in Chapter 2, used the consolidation experience to take the control in her life to another level.

CASE STUDY: SANJEETA TAKES CONTROL

'I finally learnt what it's like to say no when all my feedback is fighting against me. Psychologically and physiologically, my body was craving rest and food. It was screaming for it. But I said no, and instead took control of my body and brought it back to balance on my own watch. This level of control felt empowering and gave me confidence to take back control in my life as a whole.

'I learnt my likes and dislikes, and my self-awareness reached new heights. I discovered my triggers, my response to stressful situations, and all the old methods of escape I'd used before came to light. But this time I didn't fall for them. Even though there was no immediate checkpoint I was working towards, my mind was in control.

'I'm a new woman. I'm a strong woman. The woman who was at the bottom of the rabbit hole was using food to try to climb out, but I found out during consolidation that it was weighing me down all along. My body is now a representation of my mind: strong and healthy.'

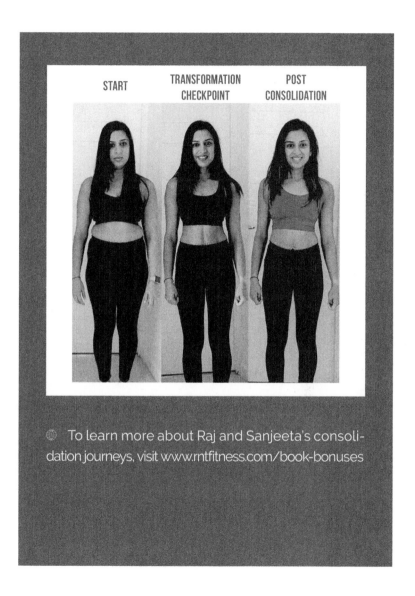

START | TRANSFORMATION CHECKPOINT | POST CONSOLIDATION

To learn more about Raj and Sanjeeta's consolidation journeys, visit www.rntfitness.com/book-bonuses

CONQUERING CONSOLIDATION

It's worrying, although not surprising, that around 80–90% of dieters regain all their lost weight, and then some. A failed or, in most cases, absence of consolidation quickly takes them back to square one, preventing them from experiencing the lasting benefits of the phases that go beyond the transformation checkpoint.

Exercise – What happened last time?

Before we move on to the investment phase, I want you to think back to the last time you dieted and ask yourself:

- How did you react at the checkpoint mark?

- Did you regain all the lost bodyweight quickly?

- What can you learn from your previous mistakes?

You may now be getting a flash of the aha moment in your head. It might even be worth rereading this chapter to let some of the tips settle in, especially after reflecting on what's happened in the past.

SUMMARY

Goal:

- Maintain the results you've achieved so far

Consolidation essentials:

- Realign with your long-term vision and why, and have a plan

- Utilise a consolidation CTP reset

- Slowly reduce the intensity of your transformation checklist

Consolidation accelerators:

- Developing meal hygiene

- Shift from an aesthetic to performance mindset

- Maintain your accountability systems

A consolidation phase typically lasts between six and eight weeks, but it can be more. You'll know you're ready to move on to the investment phase when you have mastered your psychological and physiological feedback mechanisms. You'll feel in control of your day, you'll have a handle on your food intake and you'll be energised to now make improvements.

When you're ready, let's start investing.

5
PHASE FOUR: INVESTMENT

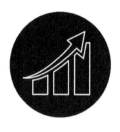

The aim of the investment phase is to work on creating further physique improvements while refining your lifestyle solutions through continued increases in your nutritional education, meal hygiene and self-awareness. This is a lengthy phase which involves the difficult task of creating a shift in your behaviour, mindset and identity to allow you to be in the shape of your life, for life.

In this chapter, you will find the term 'lifestyle solutions' used in two ways. For more clarity on the different ways I use this term, please visit the RNT glossary at the end of the book.

A LESSON IN AN AUTO RICKSHAW

A few years ago, I was in an auto rickshaw with my father in Mumbai when the driver took a risk. Turning suddenly, he sneaked in front of a moving car and just about managed to avoid crashing. While near crashes are not uncommon in the intense traffic of Mumbai, this one felt too close. So close that the driver turned around and said something to us in Hindi.

I asked my father what he'd said, and my father's answer was, 'You always need to keep moving forward. Stay still and you'll get hit.' I pondered on that statement for a while as we drove, and then asked my father what he thought of it.

'Many young auto rickshaw drivers have a dream to make enough money to leave the job and start a business for themselves. Their tenacity, hustle and drive are quite something. They see driving an auto rickshaw as a game to develop the killer instinct that may or may not carry them along their path.'

As we arrived at our destination, we tipped the driver the equivalent of the fee for the journey in the hope he'd be able to double his takings again in the future. He expressed gratitude, and then drove back into the sea of traffic to take another step towards his goals.

Later on that evening, I was journaling about the event, and as I was writing, I started to think of the concept of stagnation. Stagnation is everywhere around us, and nowhere is it more relevant than in the transformation journey.

Once you've mastered the tip of the mountain, you can invest in making lifestyle improvements to achieve your ideal physique and keep it. The problem is, after getting into the shape of your life, you may become content and flounder. Complacency can kick in and stagnation will rear its ugly head.

This is a risky place to be. Despite mastering the consolidation phase, you're still at a high risk of spinning your wheels and slowly declining under the pretence of maintenance.

Stay still and you'll get hit. It happens all the time, which is why the investment phase in the RNT Transformation Journey is where the real work begins. Everything you've achieved so far is to prime you for what's to come.

Being in the shape of your life, for life, is not about stagnation past the checkpoint. It's not about maintenance. The investment phase is where you make internal shifts in your behaviour, mindset and identity to continue building on the productive work you've done so far. It's where you create a version of yourself that can stay in shape year-round, no matter what happens in your life. It's the ability to have complete control of your body and make improvements at all times in some capacity.

In this chapter, I'm going to go through all the parts of a successful investment phase. Traditionally, this phase has been about lengthy periods of muscle building, and I agree that this is what the overarching focus should be. But it goes deeper than that. It presents a time to address your previous dieting failures and continue the work you started in the consolidation phase, building your nutrition education, meal hygiene and self-awareness.

It all starts with knowing what you want, understanding the type of investor you are, and then utilising the four investment accelerators to help you enjoy the best possible returns. Let's begin investing.

WHAT DO YOU WANT?

Every investment phase is different. As you go through this chapter, you'll learn how many directions you can take it in. You've come a long way since the beginning of the journey, and the first question you need to ask yourself is, 'What do I want?'

This phase is about upgrading yourself to version 2.0. Before going any further, take your journal out. I want you to spend time reconnecting with your why behind your why and your previous failures with mastering your body. Use these questions to guide you as you reflect, reframe and reset:

- Now that you're in the shape of your life, what do you want next in this journey?

- Where have you gone wrong in the past?

- Who do you want to be and what will you identify as?

- Is there any muck still remaining that you need to work through to eliminate destructive old habits for good?

- What benefits outside of the physical gain do you want to continue to experience?

- What do you want to learn about your body?

After going through these questions, you may have more circulating in your head, such as:

- How do you maintain what you've built more easily?

- How do you improve your physique to look even better?

- How do you prevent yourself from going back to your old ways?

- Do you need to eat this strictly and perform this much activity for the rest of your life?

- How do you sustain your physique while enjoying your food and life?

- How can you experience the life benefits of being healthy, lean and strong without being on a plan?

- What makes your body thrive?

The answers to these questions is where the value of the investment phase lies. If you want the new house you've built to withstand all conditions, you need to invest with an open and long-term mindset.

THE INVESTMENT CONTINUUM

You have two choices. The first step of this phase is determining how you want to invest. The journey unravels in two ways, revealing two types of investors:

1) The lifestyle solution. This type of investor will be someone who's always been overweight in the past, worked for years to get leaner, failed many times and now wants to learn how to stay in shape for life. A pure lifestyle solution is about refining your structure, strategy and systems so that when life gets in the way, you can work around it. It's about being able to maintain more easily, which is a goal in itself and completely different from stagnation. Being able to stay in shape year-round requires self-improvement and a change in your behaviour, mindset and identity. You have to act, think and identify as a lean, healthy person.

2) The muscle builder. This type of investor will want to focus heavily on strength and muscle. For men, they'll want to fill their T-shirts, whereas woman may want to develop their curves. The pure muscle builder will understand that they have carried far less muscle tissue and held on to more body fat than they believed they had. In an investment phase, this person will be all about setting personal records on the food plate and in the weight room, embracing the fluff of some extra body fat and thinking long term to lay down a bigger and better foundation for the future.

In the context of the house build, the lifestyle solution is about buying better furniture, upgrading the appliances, plastering the walls and making your existing house as future proof as possible, while the muscle builder will be thinking extensions, planning permits and conversions. It may be tough to deal with for a while, but the long-term gain is a house with more space, comfort and value.

You may find yourself resonating with both types of investors. Both link and feed off each other, but how you determine where you fall on the continuum between the two will depend on your psychology, background and long-term goal.

WHAT TYPE OF INVESTOR ARE YOU?

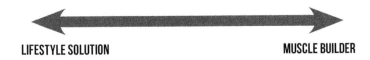

LIFESTYLE SOLUTION   **MUSCLE BUILDER**

Examples include:

- Someone who has failed multiple times on diets, spent years yo-yoing and now wants to know how to keep their new body year-round while living their life will be on the far left.

- A woman in her late thirties with kids may have a goal to stay in great shape but get as strong as possible. She'd be in the middle, slightly to the right.

- A guy in his twenties who's finished the process phase unhappy with his size will be on the far right of muscle building.

- Someone in their forties and in the shape of their life may be more focused on maintaining condition to optimise health. They'll accept slower levels of muscle growth and be more skewed to the left.

- Someone who's finally got into shape after years of trying and now wants to make further improvements to their physique while staying in good shape will be right in the middle.

Where you fall on the continuum will continue to develop as you go through your journey. How you train won't change, as you'll always be focusing on improvement. What will change is how you manipulate your body composition through nutrition and day-to-day activity.

Everyone will be somewhere along this continuum. Somewhere around the middle, maybe a little to the right, would be the position to take the first time you go through an investment phase. That's the most popular choice and the ideal sweet spot. If you're too far on the left the first time round, you may grow frustrated from the lack of tangible external gains.

Ultimately, it all comes back to what you want your version 2.0 to be. Think back to the answers you wrote down to the chapter questions to give you a better idea of where you are.

INVESTMENT ACCELERATORS

Wherever you fall on the continuum, there are four investment accelerators you'll need to upgrade to your version 2.0:

- Lifestyle management

- Performance indicators

- Health optimisation

- Autoregulation

How you approach each of these will depend on where you fall on the continuum, so keep that in mind as you read on.

LIFESTYLE MANAGEMENT

As you've gone through this journey, your 3Ss will have developed in each phase. In consolidation, you used a CTP reset to keep you on track before opening up the 20% zone, where you experiment with new foods, situations and scenarios. This 20% zone flows smoothly into this phase, as you now want to use your learning to set up your lifestyle in a way that aligns with your long-term goal. What may have worked in the lead up to your transformation checkpoint won't always work long term. Creating this change in understanding will help you as you continue to master the second half of the equation for being in the shape of your life, for life.

Wherever you are on the continuum, you need to picture your ideal week with regards to social eating, alcohol (if applicable), training and the number of steps you take, and then reverse engineer the process to your daily routine. Ask yourself:

- What is your ideal frequency of social meals out?

- What is your ideal alcohol intake without going over the top?

- What is your ideal training frequency and time spent on individual sessions?

- What is a good step target for you to achieve without it becoming a burden?

Before you get carried away, the answers need to be realistic and in line with your goals. Your actions have to align with what you want or I'd be selling you a dream. I wish I could give you the formula for enjoying unlimited meals out with a bottle of wine while barely having to move, but I'm afraid I've yet to find that missing piece. Instead, this component of investment is about understanding what works for you and what's realistic for your lifestyle. You then create the rules and strategies to fit in with your long-term vision.

Using your answers, compare them to what you want your version 2.0 to be and ask yourself if they align. If they don't, what do you need to change to allow alignment?

For example, let's say your goal is to be lean year-round while living your life to the fullest. If you're not willing to do 10–15,000 steps a day, train three to four days a week, control your portions when eating socially and limit alcohol to one to two drinks once or twice a week, you may need to rethink what you want.

When you find alignment, create daily rules. They can be anything, but they need to be the framework of your investment 3Ss. They are daily non-negotiable commitments that are decision free and have in-built precursors to allow you to execute on a daily basis. Think of this as your investment CTP reset.

For example, you could commit to:

- Always eating a protein source with each of your three meals a day

- Always having your first meal at 11am

- Always drinking 4 litres of water a day

- Eating the same meals Monday to Friday

- Going for a sixty-minute walk every morning

They'll be individual to you, but creating these rules will have a domino effect on how you live a healthier, leaner and more productive life long term. Rules are critical to making your journey sustainable while being flexible to different environments.

Living by your rules allows you to build the details of your investment transformation checklist (training, nutrition, steps, sleep and water) around your lifestyle with ease. A word of warning, though: living by your new rules in an investment phase with no looming transformation checkpoint is a task in itself. It requires an identity shift. To live a healthy, lean and productive lifestyle, you have to rewire the old behaviours which led to your trigger and the associated muck that we explored in Chapter 1.

A SHIFT TO A LEAN LIFESTYLE BEHAVIOUR

In the weeks, months or years building up to your trigger, you're likely to have been in an internal state of chaos and emotion. Poor lifestyle behaviours are almost always triggered from a place of distress. This can apply to any of the common triggers: relationships, work, insecurities and an overall lack of control. A lack of control can signify any area of your life that is falling behind. It could even be a state of boredom that you've entered from insufficient stimulation or fulfilment in those areas.

Either way, the physical is a representation of the mind. In the build-up to your journey beginning, the trigger and muck hidden deep inside of you will have created escapist behaviours destructive to your health and wellbeing, for example lack of movement, uncontrolled stress, inadequate sleep, alcohol abuse and poor dietary habits.

On the way to your transformation checkpoint, you have a clear, tangible short-term goal in front of you. While you'll have worked on your internal state from the beginning and throughout this journey, there's always a danger of old habits, behaviour patterns and routines creeping back in. Where I see this happen most is in the investment phase where the 20% zone often opens up a can of worms and exposes the work you still need to do. This is why many struggle with the second half of the equation. Even after a successful consolidation phase, it's so easy to fall back without an internal identity shift.

When you're envisioning your version 2.0, you reconnect with why it's important and use the why behind your why exercise to help drive the conclusion. This why has to be constantly reinforced so that when you're in familiar uncomfortable positions, such as at work events, social occasions or family functions, you're able to stand by who you are and who you want to be. Your old social norms or crutches shouldn't come to the surface. Instead, be confident you're on the right path and remain self-aware in the moment to make the correct decision.

This is a tough pill to swallow for many. It requires objectivity and accountability from a trusted source to decipher whether you're being true to yourself or not. The line at this stage is grey as you balance reduced rigidity in your 3Ss with your desire to build a normal lifestyle solution you can carry forward.

CASE STUDY: SURAJ'S MINDSET SHIFT

A client, Suraj, is a great example of this shift in mindset. For eighteen months, his why was driven by a desire to focus on himself and regain control of his life after the breakdown of his marriage. Despite running multiple businesses, travelling on a monthly basis and having regular social events, he kept his why at the forefront. Any potential derailing was always curbed by the goals he'd set himself and the 3Ss he'd put in place to get there.

After losing 25 kg, turning his life around on the way to his transformation checkpoint and mastering consolidation, he entered a frustrating period of wanting to have his cake and eat it. He struggled to fit in socially, where his friends and family were still indulging in the same damaging habits he'd previously joined in on, but he'd now been exposed to a whole new way of living. The problem was his environment was creating triggers of the past, forcing old behaviours, and with no immediate checkpoint, he was struggling to make good decisions.

Since identifying this issue, he's worked on why this was happening. Poor meal hygiene was a contributing factor. From a young age, he'd been wired to eat quickly, finish everything on his plate and not think about it any further. As he went past the transformation checkpoint, his need to follow a precise meal plan or calorie target diminished, so his sense of what he was eating in a social environment was only his own.

Suraj's first port of call was to heighten his self-awareness around food and tune into his body's hunger and satiety feedback mechanisms through all the meal hygiene practices explained in Chapter 4. The second step was to reflect on his previous struggles prior to starting his journey. I wanted him to reconnect with his triggers and the internal chaos and distress he was in. He needed to understand that the daily behaviours he used to have both came from these dark places and continued to feed them. It's a vicious cycle.

The final step for Suraj was to bring this all together and complete the rewiring. This came back to the question: 'Who do I want to be and what will I identify as?' This meant banishing the old 90 kg person he used to be and understanding that if he wanted a lifestyle solution to stay a healthy, productive 65 kg year-round, he needed to shift his identity permanently. He had to think, act and identify as a 65 kg person.

⊕ To dive into Suraj's life-changing story, go to www.rntfitness.com/book-bonuses.

This shift in mindset is always a tough task, but it helps you to look past the twenty minutes of pleasure that you may get from overeating, drinking too much, choosing TV over movement or skipping sleep for Netflix, bringing you right back to the place of battle your mind was in. It takes you to the lonely moments when there's no one around but you with the distress you're feeling. At the same time, you focus on the incredible benefits outside of the physical you've experienced so far, remembering just how good it feels to be in control.

If you know what you want, it makes every decision easy and temptation trivial. When you're next out with your friends and your old self would have devoured alcohol like the rest of them, your new self will be confident enough to say, 'No, I'm fine with my one drink. I'll enjoy this one and be good.'

That's the difference creating a behaviour system that allows you to stay lean year-round without slowly going back to your old self makes. Remember, if you don't rebound immediately, there's a high chance you will in the next one to three years. You have to rewire yourself.

ENVIRONMENTAL REFLECTION

Your mind may be racing right now, or you may have had your aha moment. Either way, I want you to take a moment to reflect here and ask yourself:

- What environments do I struggle to maintain my new lifestyle in?

- Which environments do I need to reconsider being a part of?

- Where do I find myself reverting back to damaging old behaviours?

This exercise requires honesty and objective thinking about which environments serve you and which ones are dragging you back down. Some of these triggering environments may be productive, just requiring you to remember who you've now become. Others will be toxic and remind you of what you don't want to go back to. Identify the environments you're placing yourself in, both good and bad, and use your new wiring to dictate your behaviour and actions. Never let it be in reverse.

PERFORMANCE INDICATORS

In the previous chapter, I introduced the concept of going from being aesthetically oriented to performance focused to create tangible targets in your investment phase. This applies no matter where you fall on the investment continuum.

If you're skewed towards the lifestyle solution, adopting a performance mindset will keep you focused in the gym and out of any ruts, while still taking the attention away from your body. The benefits mentally are immeasurable here. You identify progression in strength and movement as important parts of your life and create a cascade in behaviours that will help support this. By valuing strength, you'll want to stay hydrated, train hard, eat well and go to sleep on time. By discarding performance, you risk bringing back old habits. How you do one thing is how you do everything here.

If you're in the middle or skewed towards the muscle builder, you need to become obsessed with your performance targets. Keep this in your head at all times:

If after twelve months you're lifting the same weights as now, it's likely you'll look exactly the same.

This mindset will force you to adopt a healthy, lean lifestyle year-round, especially if you tie in the accountability reaching these targets brings with it. You can't go drinking beer until 3am if you know you need to set a squat record in the morning. You can't skip your nutritious breakfast for junk food if you know you have to bench press heavy weights in the evening. A performance mindset keeps you focused in all areas of your life, which can spill over to greater productivity at work, a stronger presence with family or a deeper 'why' behind your reason for being on this journey.

Here's how to do this. Pick one to two exercises from each of the categories listed that you can perform safely and with perfect technique. With each, I've given examples of potential lifts.

- Upper body press

    ▶ Incline barbell press, dips, military press, flat dumb-bell press

- Upper body pulling

    ▶ Bent over row, chin-ups, one arm rows, lat pulldowns

- Leg dominant variation

    ▶ Barbell squat, split squats, leg press, machine squats

- Hip dominant variation

    ▶ Conventional deadlift, dumbbell Romanian deadlift, lying leg curl, hip thrust

When you start consolidating, you're going to be feeling the fatigue and tiredness of the grind. What you're likely to want to do is wait out the fourteen- to twenty-one-day consolidation CTP reset, and then test your five to eight rep maxes on each of your chosen indicator lifts. After this, take 20% off the loading, push the reps up and slowly work your numbers up until you enter the investment phase.

Your goal now is to progressively push these numbers as high as possible while maintaining perfect form over the next twelve months. A good aim is 10–20kg on any particular lift. Keep a log book, track your lifts and make sure that when you look back each month, you're seeing progress. To increase focus, break it down into six- to twelve-week blocks and set yourself tangible short-term targets.

HEALTH OPTIMISATION

Armed with a new identity and a performance mindset, you have the perfect opportunity to optimise specific areas of your health. The core three are:

- Sleep

- Stress

- Digestion

Whole books and courses have been written on each, so I'll leave you with the most bang-for-your-buck information you can implement immediately. Improvements in each will have a positive domino effect on all areas of your lifestyle and wellbeing.

SLEEP

Sleep is the most underrated tool of transformation. It helps with everything: concentration, mood, appetite regulation, cravings, cognition and energy. It's the best medicine, and if you can get it right, you'll make every phase of your journey easier.

Here are my favourite tips for good sleep:

- Aim for seven to eight hours per night

- Wake up at the same time daily (or near enough)

- Don't hit snooze

- Get sunlight in the morning

- Train early in the day

- Avoid caffeine ten hours before bed

- No screens or electronics sixty minutes before bed

- Brain dump at night and plan your next day

- Relax

- Set an alarm to signal it's time to go to sleep

STRESS

Stress, whether mental or physical, is all the same. Your body knows no different. It perceives stress from work, relationships, commuting, dieting and training equally, and only has a limited capacity to handle it.

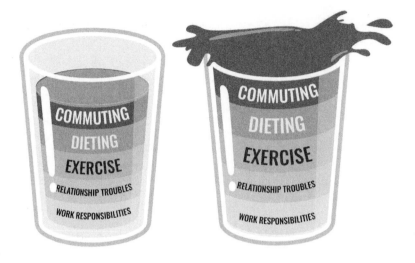

If you're not managing your stress, you will find it difficult to adopt your new identity and build the associated long-term lifestyle solutions. It'll affect your sleep, hormone production, digestion and immune system. This can be tough to monitor.

Here are six signs of an overflowing stress cup:

- You're fatigued in the morning and throughout the day

- You're wired at night, despite being tired

- You're struggling to stay asleep

- You're always sick

- You constantly experience cravings for sugar, salt and calorie-dense foods, ie you're stress eating

- You're anxious and on edge

Eye opening, right? In the busy world we live in, stress management is critical.

I asked RNT's busiest clients what strategies they like to use to combat stress. The twelve most common answers were:

- Control who and what you allow into your life. If you can't control it, don't worry about it.

- Cut down your to-do list and learn to say no.

- Create structure in your day and week. I've always loved author of *The One Thing*[11] Gary Keller's motto of being a 'maker in the morning and a manager in the afternoon'.

- Manage your screen time and don't be reactive to your phone when you wake up.

- Take at least one day off all work (and screens) per week.

- Use training as your outlet.

- Journal.

- Meditate.

- Schedule more fun time with family and friends.

- Go for a walk outside.

- Sleep more and have more sex.

- Eat wholesome, quality food on a daily basis.

---

11   Keller, G; Papasan, J (2014) *The One Thing: The surprisingly simple truth behind extraordinary results.* John Murray Learning.

DIGESTION

Maintaining a healthy gut is linked to a strong immune system, high levels of cognition and overall performance. Over 70% of your immune system is in the gut, as well as a high percentage of your neurotransmitters, including the feel-good hormone serotonin. The impact of poor gut health extends beyond the scope of this chapter, so I want to focus on one vital point.

As you begin to experiment in the 20% zone, you need to pay attention to trigger foods, both cravings and those that don't digest well. If you feel any of these after eating a specific food, you may need to reconsider your option:

- Bloating or gas

- Brain fog, poor cognition or tiredness

- Joint pain, aches or stiffness

This takes trial and error, but the benefit is you'll know which foods you digest well, and which ones to avoid even if they taste good. By default, you'll reduce your options when in social settings and be able to make choices that suit your body without any cravings or triggers.

AUTOREGULATION

Of the four investment accelerators, this is the toughest one. But it's the real moneymaker for any lifestyle solution and a critical skill to learn over the years to have the master key to your physique. It requires coaching, objective feedback, education, self-awareness and an ability to communicate so that you can learn exactly what makes you tick.

Autoregulation refers to being able to manipulate your nutrition, training and activity based on reading your short-term biofeedback (ie your energy, mood, bodyweight, body composition, strength, etc). It takes practice, and it's something I see only RNT's long-term clients achieve.

For this book, I'll be focusing on autoregulating your nutrition when in social environments, an area many struggle with. This starts with understanding the dieter's journey and seeing how it's developed through the phases so far. During each phase, your level of nutritional education will improve.

Here's a recap on what you've learnt so far:

- **Phase one: CTP – set meal plan**. Use a set meal plan to limit decisions and create structure in your diet, while learning about the foods you're eating.

- **Phase two: process – art of the buffer**. Follow a set meal plan approach for the most part with any flexibility planned beforehand. Buffering can be useful here to manage social occasions while staying on track with your short-term goals. This will introduce new foods into your database to learn about.

- **Phase three: consolidation – 20% zone**. After the CTP reset, adopt the 80:20 rule to experiment with new foods, strengthen your meal hygiene and build out your nutritional database further.

- **Phase four: investment (so far) – adopting a new identity around food**. Based on this chapter so far, make identity shifts in social food scenarios, learn more about which foods work for you and continue to develop meal hygiene.

BUILDING THE EDUCATION DATABASE FURTHER

In phase one of this journey, you'll have become accustomed to weighing your food to the gram. It's important to understand that this isn't some form of obsessive disorder when it's done at the right time. What it gives you is an invaluable expanded nutritional knowledge base and portion control, and it teaches you how your body responds to food. How else will you know what 50 g of rice looks like, or just how little 15 g of peanut butter actually is?

Weighing food is the first step in educating yourself. By the time you reach the investment phase, you will have built up a strong nutrition database. This education is one of the best investments you can make. Not gaining knowledge and being ignorant around food values and content will hinder all the potential benefits and prevent you from being able to make sensible choices when you're living life. What you'll gain from this is an ability to close the gap between your perceived value and a meal's actual nutritional value. It'll enable you to eyeball what's on a plate and get it close to 100% correct.

It's now time to accelerate your education and build your nutritional database further. Here's how:

1. **Knowledge acquisition.** This is where you add in new foods you have no experience of. You'll weigh them out, factor them into your diet using a food tracking app or tool, and take note of the portion size.

2. **Education acceleration.** When you're out in the next few weeks, order that food and understand that it'll contain roughly X calories.

3. **Repeat**. If you repeat steps one and two over four to six months, you'll gain enough education to be able to guestimate the calorific value of around 60–80% of your food and maintain your weight.

Think of this as learning the ropes at home, and then testing it in the real world. Each time you go through the process, you'll raise your education baseline and build your database. Your guestimation ability will improve and your 20% zone will become more stringent. You'll be able to gradually move away from rigid tracking and measuring to autoregulating your intake in different environments.

Here's where it gets interesting. If you combine your ability to guestimate with rules, strong meal hygiene, an identity shift, changed social behavioural patterns, a clear long-term picture of where you are heading and why, you'll be in a highly favourable position to create a lifestyle solution that works for you. This education process is the secret sauce to getting into the shape of your life, for life.

CASE STUDY: LIVING THE REAL-WORLD LIFESTYLE

Nim and Sonayna are a typical newly married couple. Their calendars are filled with social events, family functions and long hours spent at work. They like to travel and enjoy food, even classifying themselves as foodies. They also love to train, know the power of the physical as a vehicle, and are both in the investment phase.

Both skew more to the right on the investment continuum. Their goals are to build muscle, get stronger and learn how to stay in good condition year-round with their busy lives – the most popular investment choice.

While neither has any issues training hard and living by their rules during the weekdays, they struggle on the weekends. They've spent years following these behaviours:

- Identifying as foodies and using this to justify overeating

- Going all out when presented with the opportunity to eat or drink in a new environment

- Being unaware of feeling satisfied versus full versus stuffed at mealtimes

- Losing all perspective of rules when in old and/ or new environments, including holidays, restaurants or being out with the boys/girls

- Using food and drink as a crutch, and often a focal point of their social environment

In previous attempts to achieve their goals, Nim and Sonayna have been classic yo-yo dieters. They'd restrict, get in shape, go back to 'normal living' and end up at square one again. This time they want to spend their investment phase crystallising the rules that they live by to achieve their long-term goals, not what their old selves, society or their social circles want them to do. This means a real shift in behaviour, mindset and identity, consisting of these changes:

- Enjoying and experiencing the actual food in social occasions through strong meal hygiene, instead of hoovering it up as fast as possible to hold on to their foodie badges

- Staying self-aware in new environments to keep themselves grounded by their rules and their vision for their version 2.0

- Understanding when they're satisfied from a meal, rather than going all out to make the most of being out

- Building connections in ways that don't revolve around food and drink

- Making sensible decisions around portion control when in restaurants and bars, and treating meals out as just another meal versus creating a week-long buffer to allow for them

The last change has been the most difficult for them, and is likely to be for most people. Buffering is a great short-term strategy for the process phase but needs to be slowly phased out from the end of consolidation. Making this a long-term lifestyle solution has relied on Nim and Sonayna being able to use sensible portion control at all times. Examples include:

- Skipping the breadbasket

- Being happy with just a main versus all three courses

- Having one glass of wine versus the whole bottle

- Sharing a dessert versus having one each

- Picking the leaner, healthier option versus going all out with a 'dirty' meal, just because they're out

Everything is a choice. Nim and Sonayna have rewired their brains and shifted their identities. They now live in a higher state of self-awareness in accordance with their rules. It's a lifestyle, not a plan.

⊕ To learn Nim and Sonayna's best investment strategies, go to www.rntfitness.com/book-bonuses.

We've all heard the term 'breaking bread'. I believe in it and know the power of building relationships over meals. The problem is that it's now become something entirely different, whereby the bread is being broken to become a crutch and a vice. It's too easy to lose ourselves in the food and forget what being with our family and friends is all about: building relationships.

Think about when you're in a restaurant or bar. What do you turn to first? Is it the drink in your hand or the basket of warm bread? It's an easy escape.

If you want to stay within a certain weight range while making progress, you have to act like it. There's no on and off switch; making a conscious decision to maintain your structure, strategy and systems in all environments is the important lesson here. You can't spend four days a week living how you want to and three days reverting to old ways; you'll only end up frustrated, spinning your wheels and slowly making your way back to square one.

It's not about being boring; it's about living by the choices, decisions and rules that work for you and serve how you feel, look and perform in all areas of life. That's what Nim and Sonayna are doing now.

Exercise: Reassess your rules and lifestyle

- Where are you not living by your rules, why is it happening and what could you change in those moments?

- How can you accommodate more of what you've learnt so far in your journey into your day-to-day living?

- What damaging old behaviours are you guilty of letting creep back in? Are you holding on to any identities that don't serve you anymore?

MINIMUM INVESTMENT PERIODS

When you're investing in the stock market, you're advised to wait a minimum of five to ten years before you'll see any tangible results. When you're investing in your body, it takes a similar amount of time to master and reap the benefits of the four investment accelerators. Retraining all the reasons why you haven't been able to stay in the shape of your life, for life, isn't a three- or six-month solution. At the absolute minimum, you're looking at two years, but I'd lean more towards the four-year mark.

This is a period that's filled with intangible gains. Psychologically, this can be tough to grasp after being programmed to think of visible results coming in six, twelve, eighteen or twenty-four weeks. The shift needs to happen in this phase to derive any real future reward. You can't expect your house to go up in value in six months. The market doesn't work like that. It will have ups and downs, but the long-term trajectory will always show a rise.

Here are some general guidelines to follow if you want to see the tangible results in your body and experience the intangible benefits of your new lifestyle solution:

- Six to twelve months = minuscule return. This is the absolute minimum length of time required, although you're not likely to see much difference.

- Twelve to twenty-four months = good return. This is a solid timeframe to start seeing changes in your physique and your behaviour patterns.

- Twenty-four to forty-eight months = big returns. This is where you'll see a real life-changing difference in how you look, feel and perform.

These timelines will be a tough pill to swallow for many. Embrace them. Don't panic if you feel frustrated at the lack of progress or feel like you're going backwards. The worst thing you can do is throw yourself back into a lengthy dieting phase unnecessarily. This isn't the time to keep dieting. Sure, mini diets have their place and can be a tool to spark new progress and maintain healthy body composition, but going for the quick sell on your new house isn't worth it.

I started this chapter talking about the perils of stagnation. Jumping into a long fat-loss diet like we did in the process phase satisfies our need for instant gratification, but it's an illusion. It's the equivalent of panicking when the market has a down period and we feel the urgent need to sell.

Don't do it unless you absolutely must. You're selling yourself short, and you'll end up with the same body as before. You'll feel like you're making progress as you go through another grind, but it's all false. It's worse than stagnation – you've wasted time. You can't get that back.

WORKING THROUGH TWELVE-MONTH CYCLES

The best investment gains come in twelve-month cycles. That's the necessary amount of time to experience all the different events that may occur in life. Through a twelve-month cycle, you'll be able to refine your lifestyle solution during holidays, festivities, birthdays, high and low stress periods at work, and anything else life throws at you. You'll understand how you act and behave in these situations, while ensuring you have the right 3Ss in place to deal with each of them.

UTILISE SHORT-TERM GOALS FOR LONG-TERM GAINS

By now, I'm sure you realise I'm not the biggest fan of goals as a primary focus. All they do is steer you on your long-term path, but you need to know where that path is leading you. Then you can use goals to serve as your checkpoints along the way.

In the investment phase, it's easy to lose focus. That's why I like to break it down into small chunks where you're focusing on one intangible lifestyle solution goal per month and one tangible performance indicator per quarter. For example, for the next quarter you may set a goal to increase your squat by 10 kg (performance indicator), while spending time connecting to your new identity (lifestyle management), journaling (stress management) and switching electronics off one hour before bed (sleep optimisation). Another example could be aiming to add 5 kg to your bench press (performance indicator) while eliminating trigger foods (digestion), chewing your food twenty times with each bite (meal hygiene) and consolidating all the new practices you've started so far.

This brings a focus to every quarter. It allows you to stack new rules, behaviours and achievements into your life that all add up as you travel on the long path ahead. If you couple this with the accountability systems you've maintained since the start, you're going to set yourself up for a big reward phase in the future.

Objective accountability in a phase where you'll need to ask yourself hard questions is essential. It's difficult to remain objective when you reflect on years of engrained behaviour that so far has only changed temporarily. Keep your accountability systems to facilitate the long-term transformation here.

ANNUAL INVESTMENT CYCLES

In the table coming up, you'll see what three investment phases may look like, depending on your profile. You'll also notice process and consolidation phases inserted twice a year for a month. These are for when you've gained too much body fat. A lengthier process phase is only to mark your entry into the reward phase, once you're happy with the muscle and lifestyle solutions you've built.

- Option #1 – aggressive muscle builder (far right on the continuum)

- Option #2 – lean muscle builder (middle, slightly skewed to right)

- Option #3 – the lifestyle solution (far left)

The main differentiator between the profiles is the extent to which you change bodyweight. What remains constant is optimising your lifestyle solutions and building your key performance indicators.

This is only a general plan of how you may want to execute the annual cycle. If you're someone who struggles to build muscle, you may wish to only use the process and consolidation phases once in the year. For those who need to spend more time working on one lifestyle optimiser, you may benefit from one focus per quarter. It's entirely individual to you.

Month	Phase	Bodyweight change			Lifestyle optimiser	Performance indicators
		#1	#2	#3		
1	Investment	+1-2%	+0.5-1%	+0-0.5%	Identity	Build
2	Investment	+1-2%	+0.5-1%	+0-0.5%	Stress	Build
3	Investment	+1-2%	+0.5-1%	+0-0.5%	Sleep	Build + test
4	Investment	+1-2%	+0.5-1%	+0-0.5%	Digestion	Build
5	Process	-2-4%	-1-2%	-0-1%	Meal hygiene	Build
6	Consolidation	0%	0%	0%	Consolidate work so far	Build + test
7	Investment	+1-2%	+0.5-1%	+0-0.5%	Identity	Build
8	Investment	+1-2%	+0.5-1%	+0-0.5%	Stress	Build
9	Investment	+1-2%	+0.5-1%	+0-0.5%	Sleep	Build + test
10	Investment	+1-2%	+0.5-1%	+0-0.5%	Digestion	Build
11	Process	-2-4%	-1-2%	-0-1%	Meal hygiene	Build
12	Consolidation	0%	0%	0%	Consolidate work so far	Build + test

Notes on the table:

- For performance indicators, 'build' refers to making general weekly progression, whereas 'test' would mean retesting the maxes that you set at the start.

- 'Consolidate work so far' refers to refining the lifestyle optimisers you've built without adding anything new.

BUILDING YOUR INVESTMENT FUND

Navigating through the consolidation phase primes you to be in the perfect position to invest in the way you want to live, feel, look and perform. There's a challenge here that goes beyond simply staying in shape or building muscle; it's about utilising a long-term mindset to facilitate the creation of a new challenge, a new identity and a new behaviour system. It's about becoming a new person.

If the process phase teaches you what's essential in your life, the investment phase is where you create solutions for the problems you've identified. It's where you reverse engineer your unique lifestyle solution and ask the challenging questions you've been working through so far in the book about what you need to do to get there.

As you build your investment fund, you start to feel the long-term benefits of having structure and discipline in your life. You learn that structure enables you to live by strong rules that magnify everything else you do in your life. This journey isn't only about the washboard stomach you may have achieved at your transformation checkpoint; it's so much more.

CASE STUDY: TOM'S INVESTMENT IDEAS

During a photoshoot, I was speaking to a client, Tom, who'd just entered into the reward phase. After looking at the raw photos, Tom said:

'People might look at these pictures and see twelve weeks' worth of effort to get into shape. But for me, that's nearly three years of effort, discipline and dedication in what's been an incredibly productive investment phase.'

Three years earlier, Tom had been a different man. As a city executive working long, stressful hours, he was the classic programme hopper who lacked focus, confidence and control in his life. After reaching his transformation checkpoint early in his journey, he wasn't satisfied with his physique. He wanted more muscle, and even had ambitions to look like David Gandy. Ultimately, he reset who he wanted to become and knew that to get there, he needed to place himself on the muscle builder end of the investment continuum.

'I thought of muscle building as an investment. I knew if I was able to pack on muscle, it'd help me achieve the physique I wanted. In turn, it'd give me a better chance of sustaining a good physique through having a bigger engine while enjoying food and life. I wasn't sure if the science stacked up, but that's what I was aiming at.

'I spent two years making steady investments. Calories, weight on the bar, reps, more calories, more weight, more reps. And repeat. In my annual investment plan, I worked in cycles of six to eight months of building, coupled with one to two months of sharpening the sword for more growth. Psychologically it was hard to see some fat gain, but legitimate performance gain and having the long-term mentality really helped.

'And guess what? The investment paid off and I cashed out with big dividends and a body I never thought I'd have. More than that, the lifestyle solutions I've worked on at the same time in the past two years (especially with regards to digestion and sleep) means I feel completely in control of my body, its feedback and where I'd like to take it next.'

Tom's story has since evolved while he's enjoyed the benefits of being in the reward phase. He's still on a path of improvement and continues to take an aggressive muscle builder stance on the investment continuum. Stagnation is the enemy, and Tom knows that seeking growth and maintaining a strong performance mindset carries over into all areas of his life.

⊕ To learn more about how Tom's investment paid big dividends, go to www.rntfitness.com/book-bonuses.

> ### Exercise: What is your investment strategy?
>
> Now you're armed with all you need to know about a successful investment phase, what is your investment strategy? Where do you plan to sit on the continuum at this stage?

A common theme running throughout the transformation journey is control. This journey is one of self-mastery, having control of your mind, body and life to think, act and perform in the way you wish to. The internal focus you have allows for the introspection you require to decide on how you plan to take control. By going through the components of this phase, you may end up discovering the missing piece of the puzzle for your long-term lifestyle solution, the second half of the equation.

When you've pondered on what you've read, and perhaps taken stock of the elusive aha moment, let's talk about how you can cash out on your investment.

SUMMARY

Goal:

- Continue improving your physique and building your unique lifestyle solution

Investment essentials:

- Deciding your position on the investment continuum: lifestyle solution versus muscle builder

- Creating behaviour, mindset and identity shifts towards what you want

Investment accelerators:

- Lifestyle management

- Performance indicators

- Health optimisation

- Autoregulation

After a lengthy period rewiring your mind and improving your body, you're ready to enjoy the fruits of your labour in the reward phase. It's time to be in the shape of your life, for life.

6
PHASE FIVE: REWARD

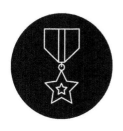

The aim of this phase is to continue improving and striving for higher levels of self-mastery through new challenges. Your mind, body and life are unrecognisable from the early stages of the journey as you enjoy being in the shape of your life, for life.

This is the holy grail. The dream house. The final piece of the puzzle. The reward phase is where everyone would like to skip to from the beginning, but few reach it. This is always for one of two reasons:

- A failed consolidation phase

- Insufficient time spent in the investment phase

Your first goal after you put this book down will be to review where in this journey you've failed before, look at the strategies required to go past it, and then utilise them in combination with your aha moment to take you on the final path to the promised land: the reward phase. By definition, the reward phase is the last part of the equation. It's when you get to enjoy the fruits of your labour and be in the shape of your life, for life.

WHAT EXACTLY IS THE REWARD PHASE?

When you're working towards your first transformation checkpoint, you spend a lot of time and energy building the structure, strategy and systems into your day to create your unique lifestyle solution. At the same time, you stay closely connected to your why, and your why behind your why. Entering the reward phase is defined by three criteria:

- You've mastered your 3Ss with transferrable rules

- You've created your unique lifestyle solution

- You have an evolving big why

You mark your entry into the reward phase by utilising these three criteria to push yourself with a new house build. This time it's a bigger, more complicated and far more expensive plan with the best fittings and furnishings on the market. You'll strive for a level of condition like never before with more muscle, lower body fat and the lifestyle solutions you've spent years investing into since your last checkpoint.

In this chapter, I'm going to walk you through the initiation of a reward phase, the new lifestyle checkpoint (the evolution from the transformation checkpoint) you'll reach and how to use reward accelerators to continue progress. This is an exciting phase to be in, and it's likely to be the one that made you pick this book up in the first place.

YOUR UNIQUE LIFESTYLE SOLUTION

Whatever answers may arise from this chapter in due course, know that by this point, you will have your unique long-term lifestyle solution. You will have a consistent set of rules you follow on a day-to-day basis that enable you to stay in the shape of your life, for life. You have a structure that serves you, systems that enable you to tick off your daily transformation checklist and strategies to allow you to work around anything that life may throw at you. Your 3Ss are locked in with the opportunity to adapt, improve and evolve while staying within the context of the rules you now live by.

Your rules should be transferrable to all environments. In fact, turn back to Chapter 2 again and scan through all your answers about your strategies and systems. These answers become automatic in the reward phase. The process is effortless. Whether you're on a night out, on a trip with friends, stuck at a networking event, in the middle of a family function or on a holiday with your children, it's all the same.

Here's an in-depth checklist for you to consider. If you can tick off all ten, you know you're ready to step into the reward phase. Many link to the accelerators we've discussed so far in phases one to four.

REWARD PHASE CHECKLIST

- ✔ Your precursors and non-negotiables are all installed

- ✔ Your day-to-day menial decisions are all automated

- ✔ You know the processes and stages required to reach a new checkpoint

- ✔ You have strong meal hygiene in all environments

- ✔ You're a master of handling social situations

- ✔ You're attuned to what you want at all times

- ✔ You can travel on holiday and return with the same body composition

- ✔ You consistently create accountability through different levels

- ✔ You're performance oriented versus only looking at aesthetics

- ✔ You're able to autoregulate feedback from your body effectively

TRANSFERRABLE RULES

I remember being in Sorrento for a week with one of the RNT team, Nathan. On the way to breakfast, he asked me what I wanted to eat.

I replied, 'The same thing I always eat – eggs on toast. If they don't have that, I'll have any source of protein with some carbs. And if they don't have any protein source, I'll fast and drink coffee till lunch.'

Luckily, the hotel had my first choice. As we were eating, Nathan asked about what other rules I live by that allow me to stay in shape year-round and transfer to any environment. Having lived the lifestyle for so long, I had made these rules automatic:

- Eat protein at least three times a day

- Maintain strong meal hygiene practices at all times

- Do something active daily, while strength training hard at least four days a week

- Fast until 10–11am

- Sleep at least seven hours a night

- Drink at least 3 litres of water a day

- Plan 60–70% of my week in advance

- Eat the same foods and meals 80–90% of the time

- Avoid any foods that trigger either digestion problems or cravings

- Start the morning with something productive and proactive that moves the needle forward in my life

This is my unique lifestyle solution and the rules I aim to live by as much as possible. There's always a need to be flexible, but these rules can guide me no matter which country I'm in, who I'm with and what I'm striving to achieve. They're transferrable and all carry benefits that cascade into every area of my life.

Part of a long-term lifestyle solution is having rules that cut out the need for decisions. If I have rules to sleep seven hours a night while starting the morning productively, that makes partying three times a week until 3am a conflicting action. If I know drinking milk triggers bad digestion, I don't need to decide when faced with all the milk-containing choices at a breakfast buffet. If I know I don't eat before 10am, that avoids the decision to wake up and eat when I'm in a new environment. There's nothing special about delaying the first meal; it's a useful rule for many to help manage calories in the day.

Living by your rules is the highest form of self-respect. Spending time defining your rules will allow you to look at your entire transformation journey as a lifestyle. This paradigm shift is what will lead to you succeeding in the second half of the equation.

CASE STUDY: STEPHEN'S RULES

Despite the birth of his two children and a high-pressure job, Stephen has continued making progress in a seamless fashion. I wanted to know the rules he maintained outside of the basic transformation checklist.

'It's been a continuously evolving process, but I'm now settling into my unique lifestyle solution. My weekly rules are:

- Remain conscious and mindful of my food, even if I don't always track it (I use my nutritional education database to carry me most days)

- Plan ahead and automate as many decisions in my life as possible to conserve mental energy for what matters most: my wife and children

- Eat whole foods 90% of the time and save experimental foods for weekends only

- Keep training, nutrition, steps, etc around family life, not instead of it – that might mean eating into sleep on some days

- Know and stay connected to my long game of building a better physique while identifying as a healthy, strong father

- Audit my life every few weeks for any insidious habits that may be creeping in and look to refine my 3Ss where I can

'In all honesty, two years on since the birth of my first child, with about 50% less time than I used to have, I'm in far better shape and have added more muscle than in the preceding ten. This is only possible because of the rules I maintain for myself.'

To find out more about Stephen's journey, go to www.rntfitness.com/book-bonuses.

WALKING INTO THE DREAM HOUSE

The direction in which you steer the development of your new dream house will all depend on where you are along the investment continuum. If you are a muscle builder, you'll mark your entry by revealing the new physique you've been building underneath the fluff you'll have accumulated.

That's exactly what I did in 2017, when I got into the shape of my life and beat all my previous conditions. This was my entry into the reward phase. To do this, I spent two years in an investment phase focusing on building muscle (once I got back on track after my failed consolidation in 2014) and learning how to operate at my best. I'd done long investment phases in the past, but never had I done one with as much focus, intensity and deliberation as this one. I was investing heavily and playing high risk.

After twenty-one weeks of dieting, I reached a new lifestyle checkpoint. I was much leaner than I'd been in 2014 with more muscle. The investment paid massive dividends. I had striated glutes, feathered triceps and I was completely shredded all round. I did this while maintaining my social life as normal and living by my unique lifestyle solution – two real game changers – and I was reaping the fruits of my labour. The combination here was key for me to enter the reward phase.

For those of you more towards the left of the continuum, your entry into the reward phase will be a little different. While you'll have built some muscle and got stronger, the majority of your focus will have been on refining your lifestyle solutions. That said, you'll still mark your entry into the reward phase with another hard dieting push. Your aim will be to go further than you did last time and execute it as effortlessly as possible. This doesn't mean it's easy, but you'll do it in a way that includes all the lifestyle solutions you've spent years investing into creating and refining.

CASE STUDY: SITAL'S JOURNEY TO THE REWARD PHASE

As a busy working mother of two young boys, Sital has always regarded her time as precious. Approaching her forties, she was in a situation many find themselves in: overwhelmed and out of control with a lack of focus and a dwindling identity. Despite spinning her wheels with different diets, programmes and plans, she was stuck in a quick-fix mindset that meant she fell prey to the four reasons for failure time and time again. It's a difficult place to be, but it can form the foundation of a powerful why once you connect to it.

When she began her journey, she went through an extended four- to six-month CTP phase to build her life by design. Her focus this time was on laying down the structures, strategies and systems that would serve her long term. She wanted to bring the focus back to herself, regain control and lay the bricks for her transformation.

There's a difference between getting into shape when you're in your early twenties with no responsibilities and when you're on the cusp of forty with two young kids and a full-time job. She reflected:

'I needed to make this work around my lifestyle and the keys for me were:

- **Crystal-clear structure.** I needed to create non-negotiables to keep everything on track, even to the point of going to bed and waking up at the same time each day, keeping workouts on the same days, coordinating with my husband on timings and maintaining a buffer of time to work around the unpredictable kids' schedules.

- **Getting my family involved.** For parts of my non-negotiables such as steps, I'd take the kids with me to the local park, get into the garden to play football and focus as much on being part of an active family as possible.

- **Continuing to connect with my why and thinking long term.** I'd failed too many times in the past by focusing on superficial reasons for change, trying quick fixes and never laying a proper foundation. This time I followed a blue-print of transformation that actually works, and I've not looked back since.'

The extra time in CTP served Sital in her process phase where she pushed through all five stages to lose nearly 15 kg and reach her first transformation checkpoint. She was almost a year into her journey, but she was in no rush. Sital was ready for consolidation where she spent four months taking the safe passage home and maintaining her bodyweight.

With a goal of building more lifestyle solutions, Sital placed herself more to the left on the investment continuum. At the same time, she remained performance driven as she reached a lifelong goal of doing weighted chin-ups.

After going through an annual investment cycle, Sital wanted to mark her fortieth birthday and entry into the reward phase with a photoshoot. Interestingly, reaching this lifestyle checkpoint brought with it far more challenges than before. She'd quit her job, launched a new business and had three holidays booked (including one all-inclusive only a week before the shoot) that meant all the lifestyle solutions she'd spent time building and refining were being tested to the max. Despite this, she celebrated her fortieth in the best shape of her life while navigating around every obstacle.

Without mastery of her 3Ss and transferrable rules in place, this wouldn't have been possible. She ticked every box required to step into the reward phase. Sital's a brand-new woman, unrecognisable from over two years ago, and is entering her forties in the shape of her life, for life.

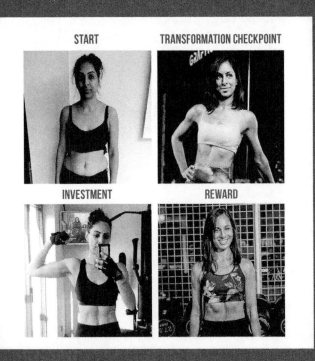

⊕ To dive into Sital's complete story, go to www.rntfitness.com/book-bonuses.

THE EVOLVING BIG WHY

Have a look back at what you identified as your triggers for picking up this book and going on this journey. I spoke about a new beginning where quick fixes and short-term mentalities are things of the past. The reward phase marks your first lifestyle checkpoint. It's where you can confidently say you've achieved the long-term vision you had for yourself on day one, along with all the necessary refinements that went into creating version 2.0 in your investment phase.

At this stage, your why will evolve yet again into something bigger than you can achieve in the near future. It will change to a way of being and will link to the mental and physical benefits you've experienced on this journey so far.

You ask yourself, 'How can I keep getting better for myself and others?' Entering the reward phase marks the moment of true transformation. While you reflect on how the physical has been the vehicle in your life, you construct your new why.

I wrote down my latest why in Chapter 1, and it has nothing to do with aesthetics. It's all about having an anchor in my day, prioritising myself and leading from the front. It's my 'me time'. I know that if I want to take care of my family, friends, relationships, colleagues, clients and the business, I have to take care of myself first. I have to be at my mental and physical best. That's my big why. The aesthetic improvement is the by-product.

If I was to take it even further, I can connect my why for the business with my why for the physical journey and marry them together. My drive for self-mastery, autonomy and future family security is all tied together with why I do what I do for my career. Being at my physical best fuels my ability to be a high performer in my career, which then feeds my even bigger why.

The more dots you can connect with your evolving why, the more engrained this journey becomes.

CASE STUDY: HOW SITAL'S AND BIRAJ'S WHY EVOLVED

If you ask Sital how her why has evolved, it follows a similar trajectory to mine.

'The journey started off as a process for improving my health and to just lose weight. But over the past two and a half years, it's evolved into a passion for fitness and a journey of self-improvement – both emotionally and mentally. I've opened my mind to form life-changing habits while understanding ways to challenge boundaries I didn't think were possible to overcome. I have a level of self-confidence and self-belief I didn't think was possible. And this journey has exposed me to resources of self-improvement that have created the best version of myself so far. It's given me a funnel to channel everything.

'Without going through the phases like I have, I don't think I'd be where I am today with my family and a newly launched business. I get asked all the time why I still train and eat well, and how I fit it around my lifestyle of running a business and two young kids. It's simple. My why is bigger than just wanting to lose weight. It's all for my family. By being my best, I make sure my family get the best of me. This is everything to me, so not taking care of myself and not striving for further self-improvement isn't an injustice to me, it's hurting my family. That's my big why.'

I remember speaking to Sital's husband, Biraj, at his second photoshoot to mark his entry into the reward phase. I sensed a shift in his behaviour. He was just different. I couldn't pinpoint it until he emailed me later on:

'I'm in the shape of my life at the age of forty. I have the structure, strategy and systems to push forward in any direction I like now, and I don't limit that to only my physical ambitions. My mindset has completely changed. I'm scoping new career opportunities, taking up new hobbies, diving deeper into my self-development, and thinking more and more about my bigger purpose here. Going through the journey has given me a platform to grow in a way I've not had before. I'm inspired, so I inspire not only my family, but also my wider circles. This excites me as I head into a decade of my life most people believe is the start of their decline.'

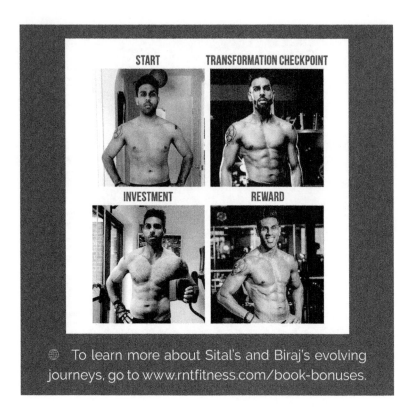

To learn more about Sital's and Biraj's evolving journeys, go to www.rntfitness.com/book-bonuses.

It's easy to get into the shape of your life. Keeping it for life and making continuous improvement is challenging, so connecting to a why that's bigger than yourself is an essential element. Before I show you some of the directions the reward phase can take you, have a think about your why. Is it big enough? Are you thinking outside of yourself?

This journey is one that walks you closer to self-mastery. It's one that allows you to regain control of all aspects of your life. It's one of self-respect and bringing the focus back to yourself. At the same time, it will allow you to positively impact those closest to you. That's the real reward, so I want you to spend a moment connecting to this feeling.

REWARD ACCELERATORS

To allow continuous improvement, there are three reward accelerators to use:

- Rebalancing priorities

- Embracing new challenges

- Recycling the journey

REBALANCING PRIORITIES

Once you've walked into your dream house and celebrated the new success, you'll start experiencing the first of many shifts and the rebalancing of your priorities with your health and fitness. What was once a top three may now be a top five. That's completely normal. Your health and fitness will bounce around in your priority list depending on your goal for the reward phase.

The difference with this phase is that no matter what life throws at you, your health and fitness will always be in your top five priorities. You'll always take care of yourself. And if you let your guard down and slip, you'll have the self-awareness to question why and course correct. That's where the power of the journaling exercises in this book come into play. It helps cultivate a level of self-awareness that brings you in tune with what your mind and body are telling you.

At this stage you need no willpower to train, eat well and reach a minimum step target. It's part of day-to-day life. It's a lifestyle, and whichever direction you take in your reward phase, you'll stick with it.

When you hear of people living the lifestyle, they're talking about being in the reward phase. I know even in my busiest times of life, training has always been an anchor in the day. If I catch my training, nutrition, steps, sleep or water levels slipping, I feel it in all areas of life. How I do one thing is how I do everything.

The physical is the vehicle. Being in the reward phase is knowing that without a focus on your physical, you're doing yourself an injustice. You'll be holding yourself back from your full potential in all areas of life.

EMBRACING NEW CHALLENGES

Once you've built the dream house, the next steps can be anything you fancy. Examples include:

- Embark on another aggressive muscle-building phase.

- Go on a slow build approach where you accept gains may come slowly, but you'd rather stay lean now. This is popular for those who've done lengthy and aggressive investment phases before.

- Maintain condition and continue to build more flexibility into your lifestyle, while refining the 3Ss you're already using.

- Learn how to utilise the physical as the vehicle to impact your highest priority in life in the most effective manner.

- Learn how to stay lean while autoregulating your trans-formation checklist.

- Maintain condition and bodyweight while focusing on relative strength (your strength-to-bodyweight ratio).

- Maintain condition while aiming to work towards the minimum effective dose of training, nutrition rigidity and general activity. This is popular for those who experience a real shift in priorities. It's about maintaining with maximum efficiency.

- Explore new sports, types of fitness and channel energy into new skills, eg gymnastics, rock climbing, powerlifting, running or obstacle course events.

The goals are endless. The reward phase is a platform to go in any direction you like; there's no right or wrong. The most popular are the first three on the list, whereby you bounce between muscle building and fat loss to continue making improvements to your physique, while upgrading your lifestyle solutions. How hard you push in either direction will depend on your new why and where you are on the investment continuum.

Ask yourself:

- How lean do you want to stay year-round? Are you happy to accept some more fluff to build an even bigger house, or are you content with a slower rate of gain?

- How much muscle do you want to build? Is the trade-off worth sacrificing leanness?

- Which body parts do you want to improve on?

- What short-term checkpoint next in your journey will best serve your current highest priority in life?

- Which lifestyle solutions need upgrading, and which ones are holding you back?

RECYCLING THE JOURNEY

Once you enter the reward phase, you're here for life. To achieve any of the new challenges you set yourself, you recycle the journey with a specific emphasis on the investment phase. This is what I like to call the reward-investment period.

When you've marked your entry into the reward phase by getting into the shape of your life, you go through consolidation again (which will be much easier this time) and start your next investment phase. There's no need to CTP again because the key criteria of being in the reward phase is to have a rock-solid foundation that never breaks. The only time you may want to utilise a reward CTP reset is when you want to realign your 3Ss and/or you're trying a new structure, strategy or system in your day.

The annual investment cycle I introduced in the last chapter is what you'll go into now. Any lengthier process phases are for later on when you've made sufficient improvements and you want to experiment in taking yourself to a whole new level of condition. This can serve to remind you of the specific benefits the grind phase can bring.

In my own example of entering the reward phase in 2017, my next step was to shift more to the left on the investment continuum. I now maintain a lean condition year-round with a good amount of muscle mass while being close to my ideal physique. My aim during this reward-investment period was to forge the key to take my physique in any direction I like. I wanted to feel in complete control of my body.

This is where many people strive to be, and it's taken me ten years to get there. That should tell you the extent of the mistakes I've made that helped form the backbone of this book. Aggressive building phases are a thing of the past for me now. I've paid my dues, deposited the pennies over the years, and since 2017, it's been all about enjoying the dividends.

CASE STUDY: TOM'S REWARDS

For years, Tom had been trying to get in shape. With high cholesterol, poor blood markers and a lifestyle of heavy drinking, fast food and long working hours, he knew his efforts were going to waste. He was the classic programme-hopping Monday to Thursday dieter who struggled with yo-yoing, lethargy and poor body confidence. He was guilty of each of the four reasons for failure and he needed to transform.

To begin with, creating and solidifying the 3Ss that worked for his busy lifestyle was the priority. He needed structure to allow for freedom, strategies to deal with all his daily challenges and systems for executing his transformation checklist. This allowed him to enter his first process phase, whereby he lost almost 15 kg to finally get into the shape of his life. He was a new man. He was no longer consumed by drink and fast food, and he was a high performer at work. His cholesterol was under control and he was ready to make this change into a long-term transformation.

After losing the weight, he wasn't happy with his size, so after consolidation, he entered the investment phase on the far right of the continuum, where he stayed for an eighteen-month period. His strength went through the roof. During this time, he was connecting with his long-term vision of who he wanted to be: lean year-round, living a healthy lifestyle and being a leader to his friends, colleagues and family.

With eighteen months' worth of pennies deposited daily in his fund, he could cash out. Tom ticked all the criteria boxes to qualify for the reward phase and he marked it with a photoshoot where he took himself into the extreme depths of the grind to surpass any previous checkpoint.

His total loss was now 19 kg from his highest weight and 20 cm off his waist. He had the physique of his dreams. Tom knew it wasn't over, though. Since reaching this new lifestyle checkpoint, he's been investing with a middle ground stance during his reward-investment phase and a focus on three goals:

- Slowly build muscle and gain strength, but stay leaner than previous investment phases

- Make his 3Ss more seamless to add more flexibility into his lifestyle

- Continue to use the physical as the vehicle to improve his relationships, career and mental wellbeing

Tom is now in the shape of his life, and it's for life. He's followed the blueprint over the past three years to develop the unique lifestyle solution that serves him, and he'll continue to reap the rewards as he now recycles the journey.

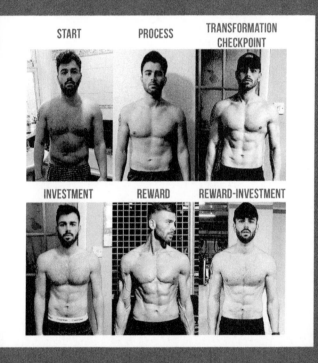

What's cool about Tom's pictures is that he's exactly the same bodyweight at his investment and reward-investment stages, which is a credit to his diligence and transformation.

◉ To go deeper into Tom's journey to the reward phase, go to www.rntfitness.com/book-bonuses.

CASE STUDY: GOING AGAINST THE GRAIN

Having reached her transformation checkpoint, mother-of-two in her forties, Minal, is an excellent example of someone with a unique investment profile that's evolved as she reached the different goals she set herself. Once she completed her first process and consolidation phases, Minal wanted to develop serious levels of strength and muscle mass. She went against the grain of someone with her background and placed herself on the far right of the investment continuum (are you noticing a common theme in those who make the best changes after their first checkpoint?).

When she asked herself what she wanted out of this phase, her thoughts at the time were:

'I like what I've achieved so far: I look and feel great, I'm more confident, and I have a structure, strategy and system to maintain this around my lifestyle. This was something I was never able to do before as I yo-yo dieted for years. I want to now be stronger with more muscle and be able to achieve an even leaner condition next time round.'

With the long-term goal laid out, Minal focused on progressive overload with perfect form while staying in a calorie surplus. Over the course of her first fourteen months of investment, she added 6.3 kg of bodyweight to go from 44.4 kg (at her leanest) to

50.8 kg. At the start of her journey two and a half years ago, Minal was exactly 50.8 kg, but have a look at the change in her body composition over that time – compare the 'start' stage with the 'investment' stage in the images below. That's smart investing.

'As the weight increased on the scales, it used to mess with my head. But looking at my physique in the mirror, I couldn't believe I was the same weight as at the start of my journey while looking like a different woman. When I think about it, this all comes down to focusing on my performance indicators. I went from leg-pressing 100 kg to 240 kg, doing lunges with 14 kg to 24 kg and adding 16 kg for weighted pull-ups, when I could previously do none.'

During this period, Minal was working through the investment phase exercises and she met all the criteria to enter the reward phase. She marked this with a six-month process phase leading into a photoshoot, where she got down to 44.2 kg and far leaner than when she had been 44.4 kg, owing to the extra muscle she'd added.

Since she's consolidated her lifestyle checkpoint, her reward-investment phase has led to her taking a far-left position on the investment continuum. She now aims to maintain condition while continuing to learn how to refine the 3Ss and lifestyle solutions that work for her.

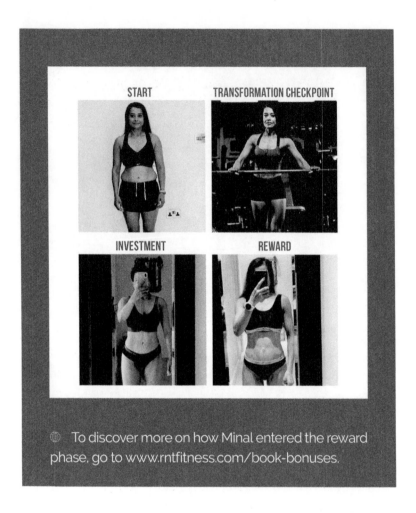

To discover more on how Minal entered the reward phase, go to www.rntfitness.com/book-bonuses.

PAY YOUR DUES

The reward will only ever be as good as your investment. The longer you invest in your version 2.0 goal, the bigger and better the reward will be. If your goal is to build 5–10 kg of muscle, you will need to go through at least three to four annual cycles of investment. That can be difficult to accept for many, which circles back to creating realistic expectations for yourself at the start. If your goal is to eat without tracking, always hold a similar bodyweight and never have to worry about dieting, then the more you invest in creating lifestyle solutions, improving your meal hygiene and understanding what works for you, the easier it'll be to reap the rewards in the future.

Don't overlook what comes before this phase. You need to pay your dues. It took me almost ten years to confidently say I'm in the reward phase. I made a lot of mistakes, both in myself and with my clients. But it's made it possible for me to now lay out a blueprint for you to get here in less than half that time. That's exciting.

I want you to question yourself more than you've ever done before. It'll be uncomfortable, but spend enough time coming up with the answers and you'll reap rewards you likely never thought were possible. You'll have a new appreciation for your own life, a new understanding. You'll be in the shape of your life, for life. You'll experience the power of the physical as the vehicle to transform you.

> ### Exercise: Make a wish
>
> If you had a magic wand to teleport you from where you are now into your reward phase, what would you wish for? What would the reward phase look like for you? What are your rules?

SUMMARY

Goal:

- Continuous improvement and self-mastery

Reward essentials:

- You've mastered your structure, strategy and systems

- You've created your unique lifestyle solution

- You have an evolving big why

Reward accelerators:

- Rebalancing priorities

- Embracing new challenges

- Recycle the journey (phases two to four)

7
BRINGING IT ALL TOGETHER

There's never a perfect time. I hope as you're reading this, you've already taken action and started your journey. If you're waiting for a clearing in your life, don't. Don't wait till Monday. Don't wait till January. Don't wait till the flowers bloom. Start now.

I've been fortunate to have seen people transform under truly remarkable circumstances. It all comes down to creating the right internal and external environment that's conducive to your success. If you lay the foundations and follow the blueprint I've detailed, you're on the right track. Don't be distracted by shiny objects, quick fixes or instant gratification. And don't compare yourself with the highlight reel of social media. That's the old way.

This book is a new beginning; a chance to rewrite your past and transform your future in all areas of your life.

THE THREE TRANSFORMATION KEYS

Over the years, I've come to see clear differences between those who succeed on the journey and those who don't.

Those who succeed get into the shape of their life – and stay there.

It comes down to the three transformation keys, which are commitment, consistency and coachability. People who hold all three are committed to the long-term journey, ruthlessly consistent over time and have a growth mindset.

Being committed to the long-term journey means having an understanding that there are two sides to the equation. There's more than just the first checkpoint. It's committing yourself to the path of self-mastery that the five phases bring. It's knowing that everything you do is part of the bigger picture, and each phase you work through links to and feeds off the others.

While you have this commitment, you know that building the momentum necessary to go through the phases requires ruthless consistency on a daily and weekly basis. It's not enough to be good for a week, then try a new thing the following week. You have to tick the boxes consistently to turn the small wins into big successes.

To accelerate your results, you need to stay coachable through a growth mindset. Adopt the identity of someone who wants to accept feedback and seek improvement. Being fixed in your old ways will lead to the same results that have failed to serve you in the past. Being growth-oriented means answering the questions in this book that may trigger you and using the answers to find the hidden lifestyle solution that's evaded you thus far.

> ### Exercise: Your transformation keys scorecard
>
> To see how you score on the three transformation keys, utilise RNT's measurement tool so you can focus on the area which needs most improvement. Before you read on, take the test at: www.rntfitness.com/scorecard.
>
> These questions will score you on your commitment, consistency and coachability, and give you a personalised report based on your answers.

REMEMBER THE CORNERSTONE

What ties the three transformation keys together is the cornerstone commitment I talked about during the CTP phase. It's making a commitment to yourself to find a solution to any perceived problem you may face. This creates an all-in mentality.

When I'm asked for the best piece of advice I'd give to anyone going on the RNT Transformation Journey, it's always the same:

Go all in. Immerse yourself into the process and jump in with both feet. Never make an excuse, never second-guess. If you're told to jump, your automatic response should be, 'How high?'

IT'S MORE THAN JUST THE PHYSICAL

As you've gone through the book, you'll have heard from the many case studies that the journey isn't only about the physical. It's a journey of self-improvement, self-mastery and self-discovery. When you bring all the elements you've been missing before into the picture, you'll create control, focus and confidence in your life.

I won't tell you this is going to be easy. It'll likely be the hardest thing you do and it'll require you to commit to your own improvement every single day. But you owe it to yourself and everyone around you. The rewards of being in the shape of your life, for life are well worth it.

DO IT FOR YOURSELF, BUT DON'T DO IT ALONE

This journey should always be about you and what you can achieve for yourself. It's not impressing others or seeking validation. That's a quick recipe for disaster.

That said, you don't need to go on this journey alone. Seek accountability, guidance and support at every stage. There's no original problem or scenario; the journey is a predictable one that will unravel in unique ways for each person. Everyone will go through the different aspects outlined in this book. While each of our bodies may process the journey in ways that require a different structure, strategy and system, the long-term path and outcome will be the same.

I always leverage the power of experts for my own journey, utilising the knowledge base of my peers and colleagues to push me to greater heights than I could achieve alone. Time is our most precious asset. If you're a busy person, you don't want to waste time making mistakes that can be easily avoided by asking the experts.

READ IN BETWEEN THE LINES

The core aim of this book is to teach you how to be in the shape of your life, for life through the five phases of the RNT Transformation Journey. But have you noticed any parallels with other aspects of your life? I've been fortunate enough to speak about the five-phase journey to experts in many different fields, and it's interesting the feedback I often receive:

- That's just how it is in business

- This applies to relationships too

- My career is on the same trajectory

If you read between the lines and understand the core principles outlined in this book, you'll be able to apply the RNT Transformation Journey to everything you do. You'll see why having the 3Ss in place for your business, fuelled by non-negotiables, automated decisions and precursors, will allow you to grow effectively. You'll understand that after the intense honeymoon period of a new relationship, you need consolidation to make sure you're both on the same page. You'll realise that if you invest heavily into your career with hours, commitment and value, you'll receive big rewards. And if you choose to opt for a career path that gives you lots of holiday and free time, you may sacrifice the financial rewards but have a better lifestyle.

When you re-read the book, apply a new lens to the phases. You might just be surprised with what you learn. Who knows, it may spark another aha moment.

YOU OWE IT TO YOURSELF

When I look back at the thousands of people my team and I have helped transform around the world over the years, there are three core benefits that run through each phase and continue to build as every day goes by:

- Control

- Focus

- Confidence

You may start from a place of chaos, distress and overwhelm, but this journey aims to help you regain control, create internal focus and generate self, body and life confidence.

One of my favourite books of all time is Victor Frankl's *Man's Search for Meaning*,[12] where he talks about how suffering can create meaning for life. His context is from the Second World War, and while I'd never compare this journey to the imposed suffering that he experienced, the wider message points to the benefit of having orchestrated suffering in your life.

The RNT Transformation Journey represents orchestrated suffering that I and many others draw meaning from every day. This self-induced personal suffering provides an internal focus and anchor to our day as it forces us to take back control of our life and rigorously audit everything. This forms a sense of liberation.

Every time you tick a box, overcome a challenge in your day and/or beat a negative emotion, you develop self-confidence.

---

12   Frankl, V (1959) *Man's Search for Meaning: The classic tribute to hope from the Holocaust.* Beacon Press.

Every time you complete your steps, nail your nutrition and/or finish a workout when life made it hard for you to do so, you build self-confidence. Every time you're able to master your emotions and the challenges in front of you, you create deeper meaning in your struggle. You build personal strength from overcoming. You become more resilient, and this shows up in all areas of your life.

The best way to build self-confidence is to keep promises to yourself, and ticking the daily checklist boxes teaches you to do this. When you're deep in the grind or you're battling consolidation and you stay in control, maintain focus and move the needle forward, you build character, self-esteem and a winning mindset. You build faith in your ability to do anything. You can make bold decisions in your career, relationships and life. You release yourself from the shackles of your past and utilise your new confidence to create a better future.

Imagine if you had the confidence to:

- Say no

- Not worry what others think

- Ask that guy or girl out

- Wear that new outfit

- Push for that promotion

- Book that trip

- Take that risk

- Banish the inner demons

- Ask for something more

- Succeed, live and be free

CASE STUDY: KRISHAN'S NEW-FOUND CONFIDENCE

Krishan experienced this new self-confidence when he lost 55 kg and took 35 cm off his waist.

'It's crazy how everything in my life came together during this journey. The physical truly is the vehicle for the greater good. From the start, I was willing to play the long game and put in the hard work. Everyone has their own demons that they have to battle with.

'For me, these started when I was young. I lost my older brother to cancer, and then I went on to have a few tough years as a teenager. This journey helped me shed those demons. What it's left me with is an unwavering self-belief, a sense of balance and a genuine appreciation of the good in my life.

'I now revel in living out of my comfort zone. I solo travelled across Asia for four months. I realised my dream of becoming a lawyer. My confidence is through the roof. And I remember one particular moment that made me realise I'd changed.

'It was at a pool party. Before I walked out to the pool, I looked in the mirror and for the first time in my life, I actually felt comfortable with what I saw. For me, it wasn't about being the leanest person. My journey (and this moment) was about liberating myself from the demons, breaking through the glass ceiling

I'd always placed above me and transcending my expectations of what I could achieve.

'Perspective is everything. For as long as I could remember, I'd been too scared to be topless around people. Picture the fat kid in the swimming pool who's so self-conscious he has to wear a T-shirt, which sticks to him and makes him look 100 times worse – that was me for some time. But there I was in a social setting with my shirt off. And all I could think was wow, this feels so strange, but great at the same time.'

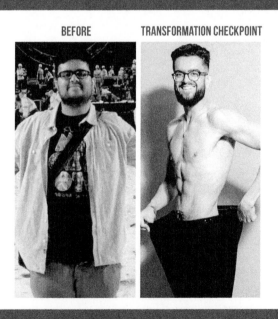

BEFORE   TRANSFORMATION CHECKPOINT

To dive into Krishan's life-changing story, go to www.rntfitness.com/book-bonuses.

This journey is the ultimate self-development tool, the spring-board for the greater good in your life. You owe it to yourself. Take action, start your journey and be ready for the physical to act as a vehicle to transform your life.

I can't wait to hear about your success story.

RNT JOURNEY CASE STUDIES

My team and I have compiled over 100 testimonials, case studies and podcasts of clients who are going through the five phases of the RNT Transformation Journey, transforming their bodies and their lives.

Head over to www.rntfitness.com/transformations to watch, read and listen to them all.

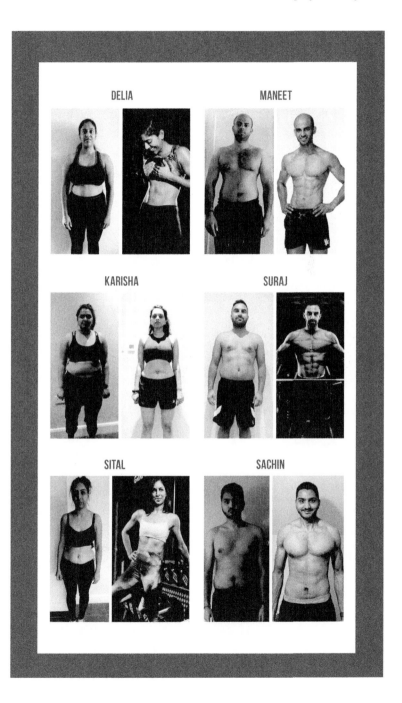

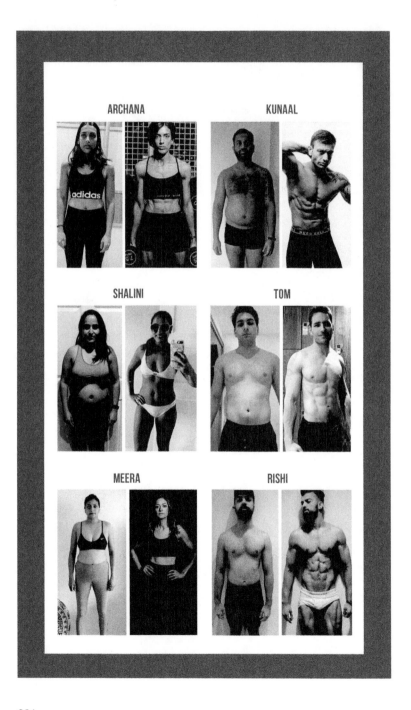

ARCHANA

KUNAAL

SHALINI

TOM

MEERA

RISHI

AFTERWORD

Congratulations on reading this book and taking the first steps on your journey to being in the shape of your life, for life. You're now well armed with all the tools, tips and knowledge required for a true transformation.

I know this book asked a lot of you. As we worked through the five phases, I asked some hard questions of you that you'll need to revisit. Find your quiet place, take out your journal and spend quality time introspecting on the questions that are most relevant to you. Be as honest with yourself as possible. Don't be afraid of the answers; that's where your growth lies.

Did you have your aha moment? Did the lightbulb shine brightly in your head? Did you discover your hidden lifestyle solution? While I speak about this journey in five phases, your aha moment will be a common theme that underpins each phase. It will be the missing piece that you have been searching for.

You'll know if you found it. Everything will start making sense. All those times you failed in the past will be valuable lessons and reference points. You'll know what you were missing and you can't wait to add it in.

If you haven't found it, that's OK. You may need to read the book again. Maybe it's a specific chapter that's calling you. Keep your eyes open; it's too important to miss.

What may strike you as you finish this book is that I've yet to mention a specific training or diet plan. There are hundreds of books on this subject. Where no book tends to venture is into how to build a unique lifestyle solution around the transformation checklist.

This is where a coach can come in as a facilitator on your journey of self-discovery. A coach mentors you through the blueprint of your individual physical transformation success, holding you accountable to ticking all the boxes that ultimately activate the vehicle and enable you to make the change you want.

I can't say how much I appreciate you investing your time and energy into reading this book. I hope it's been worth it and that you've gained value, both in the short term and for years to come. Thank you for coming along on the journey with me, and if I can ever be of assistance or answer any questions you may have, I can be reached at akash.vaghela@rntfitness.com. I look forward to hearing from you.

Plus...

If you've gained value from reading this, I'd be so grateful if you could leave a review on Amazon, so that more people can learn about the teachings of the book.

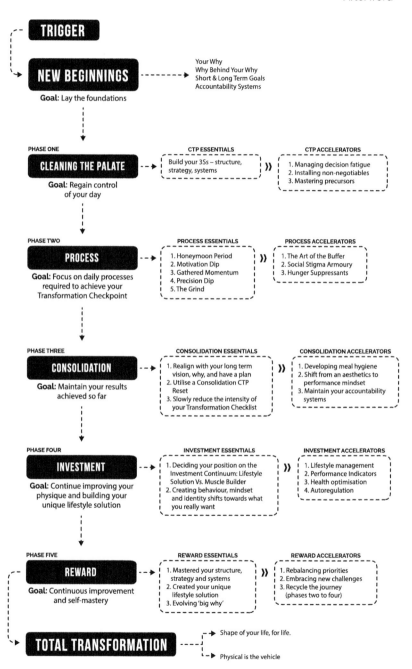

THE RNT TRANSFORMATION JOURNEY: THE FIVE-PHASE METHOD TO BEING IN THE SHAPE OF YOUR LIFE, FOR LIFE

RNT RESOURCES

Here are a few resources to help you transform into the shape of your life, for life. To access them, go to www.rntfitness.com/book-bonuses.

Special bonus: To help you kickstart your journey, I'm offering some free special bonus downloads for you, including printable worksheets and a starter plan.

Education resources: For the most relevant articles, podcasts and videos to help accelerate your education. You'll be able to access all the case studies I've mentioned along the way.

RNT transformation scorecard: To score yourself on the three transformation keys. You'll receive a personalised report with actionable tips on how to improve your score and prime yourself for transformation.

RNT online coaching: To learn how you can use the power of one-to-one coaching and accountability to guide you through the RNT Transformation Journey, go to www.rntfitness.com/services or email my team on info@rntfitness.com.

REFERENCES

I've made reference to some brilliant books, minds and research:

Baumeister, R F; Tierney, J (2012) *Willpower: Why self-control is the secret to success.* Penguin

Bloem, C (2018) 'Successful People Wear the Same Thing Every Day'. www.inc.com/craig-bloem/this-1-unusual-habit-helped-make-mark-zuckerberg-steve-jobs-dr-dre-successful.html

Clear, J (2018) *Atomic Habits: An easy and proven way to build good habits and break bad ones.* Random House Business

Coelho, P (2017) 'Discipline and freedom are not mutually exclusive' [Facebook post] 23 February 2017. www.facebook.com/paulocoelho/phot os/a.241365541210/10154880056531211/?type=1&theater

Fogg, B J (2019) *Tiny Habits: The small changes that change everything.* Virgin Books

Frankl, V (1959) *Man's Search For Meaning: The classic tribute to hope from the Holocaust.* Beacon Press

Godin, S (2007) *The Dip: The extraordinary benefits of knowing when to quit (and when to stick).* Piatkus

Goggins, D (2018) *Can't Hurt Me: Master your mind and defy the odds.* Lioncrest Publishing

IMARC Group (2019) 'Weight Management Market: Global Industry Trends, Share, Size, Growth, Opportunity and Forecast 2019–2024'. www.imarcgroup.com/weight-management-market

Keller, G; Papasan, J (2014) *The One Thing: The surprisingly simple truth behind extraordinary results.* John Murray Learning

Lally, P; van Jaarsveld, C H M; Potts, H W W; Wardle, J (2010) 'How Are Habits Formed: Modelling habit formation in the real world'. *European Journal of Social Psychology*

RNT GLOSSARY

3Ss:

- Structure – how you set your day and week up for success

- Strategy – how you work around life while striving towards your goals

- System – how you plan to execute what you need to action on a daily and weekly basis

20% zone. When you adopt the 80:20 rule with your nutritional rigidity and use the 20% to experiment with new foods and increase your education.

Accelerators. The tools you can use to help navigate through each phase to maximise your chance of success.

Buffer. The act of reducing calorie intake or increasing calorie expenditure to create room and account for a higher calorie intake when in social environments.

Embracing the fluff. The acceptance of the inevitable additional body fat that comes with aggressive muscle-building phases, with a view to making significant changes past your first transformation checkpoint.

The equation:

- Both sides of the equation is getting into the shape of your life, for life

- First half of the equation refers to getting into the shape of your life

- Second half of the equation refers to the 'for life' part

Guestimation. Your ability to calculate the nutritional values of different foods without knowing the contents or methods of cooking.

Investment continuum. Understanding where on the spectrum you approach your investment phase from, whether it's as a lifestyle solution or muscle builder.

Lifestyle checkpoint. It's the moment you enter the reward phase in the shape of your life – the evolution from your transformation checkpoint.

Lifestyle solution. This term is used in three ways throughout this book:

- **Create your long-term lifestyle solution.** This refers to the second half of the equation. It's having your 3Ss and rules in order so you can be in the shape of your life, for life.

- **Build your lifestyle solutions.** This refers to all the different accelerators, tools and strategies taught throughout the journey that allow you to be in shape while living your lifestyle, for example meal hygiene, decision fatigue, identity shifts, 20% zones, etc. It's everything this book teaches to facilitate permanent change.

- **Take the lifestyle solution option.** This refers to being on the far left of the investment continuum. If you take this approach, your goal will be to learn how to stay in shape year-round. Your focus will be on behaviour, mindset and identity change.

Meal hygiene. Your ability to use healthy eating practices at meal times to promote satiety, enjoyment and a positive relationship around food.

Muck. The deep-rooted distress or struggle that's caused poor lifestyle choices in the past.

The muscle builder. This refers to being on the far right of the investment continuum. If you take this approach, your goal will be to add as much strength and muscle as possible.

Nutrition database. Your education around food quantities, values and contents.

Precursors. The small actions you take moments prior to bigger actions that make execution easier. They're the decision before the decision.

Tip of the mountain. The period of time from the start of the grind in the process phase to the end of consolidation. The summit refers to the transformation checkpoint.

Transformation checkpoint. The moment you're in the shape of your life for the first time in the journey.

Trigger. The specific moment, feeling or event that makes you realise you need to transform.

ACKNOWLEDGEMENTS

I was deep into the #VaghelaGrind when I realised it was time to start writing this book. To see it come to fruition is a special moment, and one I wholeheartedly know wouldn't have been possible without the incredible support team I have around me.

First and foremost, I want to thank my clients, friends and guinea pigs who've trusted me enough over the past decade to test my theories and experiment, ultimately empowering themselves to transform their bodies and their lives for the greater good. Without you, this book wouldn't have been possible. Specifically, I want to thank those of you who've graciously allowed me to tell your stories in case studies, including Shyam, Maneet, Sanjeeta, Archana, Roshni, Akash, Dhinil, Diksesh, Sachin, Raj, Puja, Tim, Kunaal, Adam, Tej, Dhaval, Suraj, Nim, Sonayna, Tom H, Stephen, Sital, Biraj, Tom B, Minal and Krishan.

To my excellent publishing team at Rethink Press, headed up by Lucy and Joe. You've made a ten-year dream come true – thank you. Special mentions go to Siobhan, for helping me plan this book by spending a whole day downloading a decade's worth of insights; Alison, for meticulously editing the final manuscript; and Kathleen, for managing the entire project.

To the people who read through the many alterations and drafts of the book, including Nathan, Puja, Raj, Tim, Shyam, Nim, Tasneem,

Tej, Chandni and my dad – thank you for your patience, your critical eye and for understanding the mission of the book. You kept me on the right track at all times.

To my inner circle of trusted friends, confidantes and consiglieres, including Shyam, Jai, Bilal, Sindu, Bhavik, Amar, Dhinil, Abz, Hari and Minil – your support and belief in me is never forgotten. I draw inspiration from each and every one of you, every day.

To all my teachers, mentors, advisors and coaches in the past decade, thank you for the guidance, wisdom and knowledge you've been gracious enough to impart to me.

Thank you to the current RNT team of coaches: Nathan Johnson, Kunal Makwana, Ben Mulamehic, Elliot Hasoon, Ivan Gavranic, Ed Pilkington, Shaneeta Malik, Ed Pimley and Samir Oukili.

Behind these facilitators is the team that makes it all possible. I'd like to thank Puja Teli, RNT's business manager, for always believing in my mission and allowing me to focus on the book; Cyleena Nieto, for your help in researching key elements; Nimalan Chandran, for always pushing me to strive for excellence; Suraj Sodha, for managing RNT's online presence and producing the incredible graphics in this book and all over the website.

A special note to Nathan Johnson, head of education at RNT, whose many thoughtful conversations, meticulous research and creative ideas have helped in the formalisation of the five-phase methodology – which we first wrote on the back of a notepad on an aeroplane to Italy. Thank you for everything you've poured into this book.

To my Ba and my sister, Roshni, thank you for allowing me to go into my shell of writing while understanding that your grandson/brother was on a mission.

To my better half and partner in crime, Chandni. Your belief in me and the support you give to everything I do never ceases to amaze me. From reading each segment of the book at every stage of the journey, to understanding when I fell asleep at 8pm from writing and editing exhaustion, to pushing me when I wanted to give up, you've been the lynchpin in bringing this book to life. Thank you so much.

And last but not least, to my parents – Dipak and Divya Vaghela – for bringing me into this world and supporting, encouraging, motivating and inspiring me to be the best version of myself on the path I've chosen. My greatest mentors. I'll never forget the sacrifices you've made to allow me to do what I do. You were the first people to believe in me and I am forever grateful.